# Ophthalmology

*Editors*

PAUL J. BRYAR
NICHOLAS J. VOLPE

# MEDICAL CLINICS
# OF NORTH AMERICA

www.medical.theclinics.com

*Consulting Editor*
JACK ENDE

May 2021 • Volume 105 • Number 3

**ELSEVIER**

1600 John F. Kennedy Boulevard • Suite 1800 • Philadelphia, Pennsylvania, 19103-2899

http://www.theclinics.com

**MEDICAL CLINICS OF NORTH AMERICA Volume 105, Number 3**
**May 2021 ISSN 0025-7125, ISBN-13: 978-0-323-81309-9**

Editor: Katerina Heidhausen
Developmental Editor: Arlene Campos

Medical Clinics of North America (ISSN 0025-7125) is published bimonthly by Elsevier Inc., 360 Park Avenue South, New York, NY 10010-1710. Months of publication are January, March, May, July, September, and November. Business and editorial offices: 1600 John F. Kennedy Boulevard, Suite 1800, Philadelphia, PA 19103-2899. Periodicals postage paid at New York, NY, and additional mailing offices. Subscription prices are USD $304.00 per year (US individuals), $910.00 per year (US institutions), $100.00 per year (US Students), $381.00 per year (Canadian individuals), $965.00 per year (Canadian institutions), $200.00 per year for (foreign students), $100.00 per year for (Canadian students), $422.00 per year (foreign individuals), and $965.00 per year (foreign institutions). To receive student/resident rate, orders must be accompanied by name of affiliated institution, date of term, and the signature of program/residency coordinator on institution letterhead. Orders will be billed at individual rate until proof of status is received. Foreign air speed delivery is included in all Clinics' subscription prices. All prices are subject to change without notice. **POSTMASTER:** Send address changes to *Medical Clinics of North America*, Elsevier Health Sciences Division, Subscription Customer Service, 3251 Riverport Lane, Maryland Heights, MO 63043. **Customer Service: Telephone: 1-800-654-2452** (U.S. and Canada); **1-314-447-8871** (outside U.S. and Canada). **Fax: 314-447-8029. E-mail: journalscustomerserviceusa@ elsevier.com** (for print support); **journalsonlinesupport-usa@elsevier.com** (for online support).

*Reprints.* For copies of 100 or more of articles in this publication, please contact the Commercial Reprints Department, Elsevier Inc., 360 Park Avenue South, New York, NY 10010-1710. Tel.: 212-633-3874; Fax: 212-633-3820; E-mail: reprints@elsevier.com.

*Medical Clinics of North America* is also published in Spanish by McGraw-Hill Interamericana Editores S. A., P.O. Box 5-237, 06500 Mexico, D.F., Mexico.

*Medical Clinics of North America* is covered in *MEDLINE/PubMed (Index Medicus), Current Contents, ASCA, Excerpta Medica, Science Citation Index,* and *ISI/BIOMED.*

## PROGRAM OBJECTIVE
The goal of the *Medical Clinics of North America* is to keep practicing physicians up to date with current clinical practice by providing timely articles reviewing the state of the art in patient care.

## TARGET AUDIENCE
All practicing physicians and other healthcare professionals.

## LEARNING OBJECTIVES
Upon completion of this activity, participants will be able to:
1. Review the vast array of visual disorders.
2. Explain how visual Impairment can be prevented in most patients with early detection and treatment.
3. Discuss the impact visual disorders have on both individuals and society.

## ACCREDITATION
The Elsevier Office of Continuing Medical Education (EOCME) is accredited by the Accreditation Council for Continuing Medical Education (ACCME) to provide continuing medical education for physicians.

The EOCME designates this journal-based CME activity for a maximum of 11 *AMA PRA Category 1 Credit*(s)™. Physicians should claim only the credit commensurate with the extent of their participation in the activity.

All other healthcare professionals requesting continuing education credit for this enduring material will be issued a certificate of participation.

## DISCLOSURE OF CONFLICTS OF INTEREST
The EOCME assesses conflict of interest with its instructors, faculty, planners, and other individuals who are in a position to control the content of CME activities. All relevant conflicts of interest that are identified are thoroughly vetted by EOCME for fair balance, scientific objectivity, and patient care recommendations. EOCME is committed to providing its learners with CME activities that promote improvements or quality in healthcare and not a specific proprietary business or a commercial interest.

**The planning committee, staff, authors and editors listed below have identified no financial relationships or relationships to products or devices they or their spouse/life partner have with commercial interest related to the content of this CME activity:**
Cynthia A. Bradford, MD; Paul J. Bryar, MD; Arlene Campos; Christopher B. Chambers, MD; Regina Chavous-Gibson, MSN, RN; Neena R. Cherayil, MD; Maura Di Nicola, MD; Jack Ende, MD, MACP; Hesham Gabr, MD; Manjot K. Gill, MD; Dilraj S. Grewal, MD; Katerina Heidhausen; J. Minjy Kang, MD; Hong-Gam Le, MD; Emily Li, MD; Andrew T. Melson, MD; Rukhsana G. Mirza, MD, MS; Ahmad Rehmani, DO; Carol H. Schmidt, MD; Akbar Shakoor, MD; Jeyanthi Surendrakumar; Misha Syed, MD; Madhura A. Tamhankar, MD; Catherine J. Thomas, MD, MHA, MS; Nicholas J. Volpe, MD; Matthew Yang, MD; Sonia H. Yoo, MD; Mike Zein, MD

**The planning committee, staff, authors, and editors listed below have identified financial relationships or relationships to products or devices they or their spouse/life partner have with commercial interest related to the content of this CME activity:**
Angelo P. Tanna, MD: consultant/advisor for Bausch & Lomb Incorporated, Ivantis, Inc, and Zeiss International

Basil K. Williams, Jr, MD: consultatant/advisor for Genentech, Inc and Castle Biosciences, Inc.

## UNAPPROVED/OFF-LABEL USE DISCLOSURE
The EOCME requires CME faculty to disclose to the participants;
1. When products or procedures being discussed are off-label, unlabelled, experimental, and/or investigational (not US Food and Drug Administration [FDA] approved); and
2. Any limitations on the information presented, such as data that are preliminary or that represent ongoing research, interim analyses, and/or unsupported opinions. Faculty may discuss information about pharmaceutical agents that is outside of FDA-approved labelling. This information is intended solely for CME and is not intended to promote off-label use of these medications. If you have any questions, contact the medical affairs department of the manufacturer for the most recent prescribing information.

**TO ENROLL**

To enroll in the *Medical Clinics of North America* Continuing Medical Education program, call customer service at 1-800-654-2452 or sign up online at http://www.theclinics.com/home/cme. The CME program is available to subscribers for an additional annual fee of USD 324.00.

**METHOD OF PARTICIPATION**

In order to claim credit, participants must complete the following;

1. Complete enrolment as indicated above.
2. Read the activity.
3. Complete the CME Test and Evaluation. Participants must achieve a score of 70% on the test. All CME Tests and Evaluations must be completed online.

**CME INQUIRIES/SPECIAL NEEDS**

For all CME inquiries or special needs, please contact elsevierCME@elsevier.com.

# MEDICAL CLINICS OF NORTH AMERICA

---

**SERIES OF RELATED INTEREST**

*Primary Care: Clinics in Office Practice*
https://www.primarycare.theclinics.com/

---

# MEDICAL CLINICS OF NORTH AMERICA

## SERIES OF RELATED INTEREST

# Contributors

## CONSULTING EDITOR

**JACK ENDE, MD, MACP**
The Schaeffer Professor of Medicine, Department of Medicine, Perelman School of Medicine, University of Pennsylvania, Philadelphia, Pennsylvania, USA

## EDITORS

**PAUL J. BRYAR, MD**
Professor of Ophthalmology and Pathology, Northwestern University Feinberg School of Medicine, Chicago, Illinois, USA

**NICHOLAS J. VOLPE, MD**
George and Edwina Tarry Professor of Ophthalmology, Chairman, Department of Ophthalmology, Northwestern University Feinberg School of Medicine, Chicago, Illinois, USA

## AUTHORS

**CYNTHIA A. BRADFORD, MD**
Professor, Department of Ophthalmology, University of Oklahoma, College of Medicine, Dean A. McGee Eye Institute, Oklahoma City, Oklahoma, USA

**PAUL J. BRYAR, MD**
Professor of Ophthalmology and Pathology, Northwestern University Feinberg School of Medicine, Chicago, Illinois, USA

**CHRISTOPHER B. CHAMBERS, MD**
Department of Ophthalmology, University of Washington School of Medicine, Seattle, Washington, USA

**NEENA R. CHERAYIL, MD**
Assistant Professor, Departments of Neurology and Ophthalmology, Northwestern University, Chicago, Illinois, USA

**MAURA DI NICOLA, MD**
Ocular Oncology Service, Department of Ophthalmology, University of Cincinnati College of Medicine, Cincinnati, Ohio, USA

**HESHAM GABR, MD**
Department of Ophthalmology, Duke University, Durham, North Carolina, USA; Department of Ophthalmology, Ain Shams University, Cairo, Egypt

**MANJOT K. GILL, MD, FRCS (C)**
Associate Professor, Department of Ophthalmology, Northwestern University Feinberg School of Medicine, Chicago, Illinois, USA

**DILRAJ S. GREWAL, MD**
Department of Ophthalmology, Duke University, Durham, North Carolina, USA

**JESSICA MINJY KANG, MD**
Assistant Professor, Department of Ophthalmology, Northwestern University Feinberg School of Medicine, Chicago, Illinois, USA

**HONG-GAM LE, MD**
Retina Fellow, John A. Moran Eye Center, Salt Lake City, Utah, USA

**EMILY LI, MD**
Department of Ophthalmology, University of Washington School of Medicine, Seattle, Washington, USA

**ANDREW T. MELSON, MD**
Assistant Professor, Department of Ophthalmology, University of Oklahoma, College of Medicine, Dean A. McGee Eye Institute, Oklahoma City, Oklahoma, USA

**RUKHSANA G. MIRZA, MD, MS**
Department of Ophthalmology, Professor of Ophthalmology and Medical Education, Northwestern University Feinberg School of Medicine, Chicago, Illinois, USA

**AHMAD REHMANI, DO**
Vitreoretinal Fellow, University of Texas Medical Branch, Galveston, Texas, USA

**CAROL H. SCHMIDT, MD**
Assistant Professor of Ophthalmology, Northwestern University Feinberg School of Medicine, Chicago, Illinois, USA

**AKBAR SHAKOOR, MD**
Associate Professor, John A. Moran Eye Center, Salt Lake City, Utah, USA

**MISHA F. SYED, MD, MEHP**
Professor of Ophthalmology, University of Texas Medical Branch, Galveston, Texas, USA

**MADHURA A. TAMHANKAR, MD**
Department of Ophthalmology and Neurology, University of Pennsylvania, Philadelphia, Pennsylvania, USA

**ANGELO P. TANNA, MD**
Professor, Department of Ophthalmology, Northwestern University Feinberg School of Medicine, Chicago, Illinois, USA

**CATHERINE J. THOMAS, MD, MHA, MS**
Department of Ophthalmology, Northwestern University Feinberg School of Medicine, Chicago, Illinois, USA

**NICHOLAS J. VOLPE, MD**
George and Edwina Tarry Professor of Ophthalmology, Chairman, Department of Ophthalmology, Northwestern University Feinberg School of Medicine, Chicago, Illinois, USA

**BASIL K. WILLIAMS Jr. MD**
Ocular Oncology Service, Department of Ophthalmology, University of Cincinnati College of Medicine, Cincinnati, Ohio, USA

**MATTHEW YANG, MD**
Ophthalmology Resident, University of Texas Medical Branch, Galveston, Texas, USA

**SONIA H. YOO, MD**
Professor of Ophthalmology, Greentree Hickman Chair in Ophthalmology, Associate Medical Director, Cornea and Refractive Surgery Department, Department of Ophthalmology, Bascom Palmer Eye Institute, University of Miami Miller School of Medicine, Miami, Florida, USA

**MIKE ZEIN, MD**
McKnight Vision Research Center, Bascom Palmer Eye Institute, University of Miami Miller School of Medicine, Miami, Florida, USA

# Contents

Incidence of cataract, diabetic retinopathy, macular degeneration, and glaucoma will significantly increase by 2050. Visual impairment can increase morbidity and mortality in nonocular disease. There are different patterns of vision loss in cataract, diabetic retinopathy, age-related macular degeneration, and glaucoma. Internists and medical subspecialists play an important role in prevention, detection, and early treatment of eye disease. Awareness of screening guidelines for eye disease as well as a basic ocular history and simple penlight examination can decrease incidence of vision loss and its impact. Visual impairment places a significant financial burden on society.

Primary care physicians see nearly half of all clinical visits, and 2% to 3% of those are for eye complaints. Taking a good ocular history is essential to establishing the diagnosis. Patient complaints fall into several categories including visual change, redness, and pain. Primary care physicians can screen for patients at risk of vision loss from glaucoma, diabetes, and toxic medication and ensure that patients have appropriate eye evaluations. Examination techniques such as direct ophthalmoscopy, evaluation of the red reflex, eversion of the upper lid, checking pupillary response, and using fluorescein to stain the cornea are helpful in evaluating patients' ocular complaints.

When prescribing medications, it is important to consider the ocular side effects of common systemic therapy as well as potential systemic side effects of ocular medications. Although not an exhaustive list of medications/classes of medications, this article does include many commonly used drugs and also provides information on some topical therapies commonly used by ophthalmologists. These ocular medications may result in systemic effects and/or alter patients' management of systemic conditions.

damage to the visual system; however, early diagnosis and treatment can prevent progression of the disease. In most cases, glaucoma is a chronic condition that requires lifelong management. This article reviews the pathophysiology, classification, clinical manifestations, diagnosis, and management of glaucoma.

Neena R. Cherayil and Madhura A. Tamhankar

 Video content accompanies this article at http://www.medical. theclinics.com.

Neuro-ophthalmology is the study of the neurologic underpinnings of vision and includes a fascinating variety of disorders that span the broad spectrum of ophthalmic and neurologic disease. This subspecialty relies heavily on accurate neuroanatomic localization and examination. This article discusses neuro-ophthalmic complaints that frequently present to the internist, including acute vision loss, double vision, and unequal pupils. It focuses on pertinent clinical features of the most common causes of these chief complaints and additionally highlights salient points of history, diagnosis, examination, and management with special emphasis on the signs and symptoms that should prompt expedited evaluation.

Basil K. Williams Jr. and Maura Di Nicola

Several neoplastic processes can involve the eye, either primarily or secondary to a systemic malignancy. The most common primary tumors of the eye include conjunctival and uveal melanoma, retinoblastoma, conjunctival and intraocular lymphoma, and ocular surface squamous neoplasia. Metastatic spread from systemic malignancies, especially of the breast and lung, also can involve the eye. A combination of ophthalmologic examination, ancillary testing, and cytologic/histopathologic evaluation leads to accurate diagnosis. Management consists of surgery, radiotherapy, chemotherapy, and immunotherapy delivered in various forms.

Emily Li and Christopher B. Chambers

The eyelids and orbit encompass intricate bony and soft tissue structures that work harmoniously in concert to protect, support, and nourish the eye in order to facilitate and maintain its function. Insult to periorbital and orbital anatomy can compromise orbital and ocular homeostasis. This article provides a foundational overview of eyelid and orbital anatomy, as well as common and key disorders that may confront internists and medical subspecialists.

Dilraj S. Grewal and Hesham Gabr

Comprehensive patient care requires an integrated approach that often includes different specialties. Of these specialties, Ophthalmology stands out with its variable pathologic conditions, unique tools, and special examination techniques, which are not part of the standard training of internal medicine or other specialties. The authors review prior studies focused on inpatient ophthalmology consultations, common reasons for inpatient ophthalmology consultation, and the recommended approach to the most common ocular complaints that could present to the inpatient provider. They also shed light on the basic ocular history and eye examination that should be obtained before requesting an ophthalmic evaluation.

# Foreword
# When to Refer

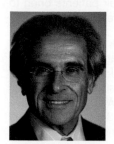

Jack Ende, MD, MACP
*Consulting Editor*

Of all the challenges faced by general internists and other primary care providers, When to Refer is among the most important. Patients present with problems that may be outside their providers' area of expertise, both diagnostically and therapeutically, and so referral to an appropriate specialty colleague is required.

In no field is this more vital than ophthalmology. As Guest Editors, Drs Paul J. Bryar and Nicholas J. Volpe in *Eye Care for the Internist* explain in their Preface, there are many reasons for this. Suffice it to say, primary care providers rely on ophthalmologists to ensure their patients are receiving proper treatment for ocular and vision problems.

But that is not to say that these internists and their primary care colleagues should not be handling many ophthalmologic complaints seen in office practice. They can and should. Moreover, these same primary care providers have a critical role to play in ensuring that their patients are receiving appropriate eye care and taking measures that can prevent blindness. Medicine is a team sport, basketball, if you will, and primary care providers need to know how and when to pass the ball, but also when it is best for them to take the shot.

In his recent book, *Think Again: The Power of Knowing What You Don't Know*, organizational psychologist Adam Grant[1] correctly points out the value of identifying the boundaries of one's knowledge. All true. But is it not also valuable to push these boundaries? I want to know as much as I can about the ocular and vision problems my patient brings to me. I want to know how to evaluate their complaints and ensure that they are receiving proper preventive care.

*Eye Care for the Internist* provides an up-to-date guide to accomplishing exactly that. Drs Volpe and Bryar, and their expert authors, have done us all a great service by bringing together in one issue what primary care providers need to know and what their ophthalmologic colleagues are able to do. Topics range from common ocular complaints that primary care providers should be able to handle, to ophthalmologic, vision-threatening emergencies. Eye problems associated with common

Med Clin N Am 105 (2021) xv–xvi
https://doi.org/10.1016/j.mcna.2021.03.001
0025-7125/21/© 2021 Published by Elsevier Inc.

systemic illnesses are covered, as are the highly prevalent ophthalmologic illnesses (eg, glaucoma, cataracts, and macular degeneration), and less common but still important problems managed by our ophthalmology colleagues, such as oncologic ocular issues. The issue also includes an article on eye problems seen on the inpatient service. All these topics are presented specifically for practicing primary care providers, who need to understand the eye and vision problems their patients bring to their attention, and when to refer. This is a valuable resource, indeed.

Jack Ende, MD, MACP
Department of Medicine
Perelman School of Medicine of the
University of Pennsylvania
5033 West Gates Pavilion
3400 Spruce Street
Philadelphia, PA 19104, USA

*E-mail address:*
jack.ende@pennmedicine.upenn.edu

## REFERENCE

1. Grant A. Think again: the power of knowing what you don't know. New York: Viking; 2021.

# Preface

# Eye Care for the Internist

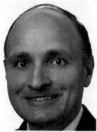 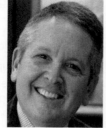

Paul J. Bryar, MD    Nicholas J. Volpe, MD
*Editors*

As a consequence of limited time devoted to eye disease in medical school, highly technical, not readily available, and unfamiliar instruments used to examine the eye, and ophthalmic progress notes that are often indecipherable to the internist, many nonophthalmologist physicians view ocular complaints and disease as impossible to evaluate meaningfully and something to refer to an eye care provider. One may think that the main goal of this issue is to unravel the mystery and shed light on an organ that is difficult to examine and has diseases they rarely encounter. Quite the opposite is true. The authors describe ocular symptoms and diseases commonly encountered by internists and medical subspecialists. More importantly, we demonstrate how internists and medical subspecialists are arguably the most important providers in preventing vision loss.

The majority of visual impairment and vision loss is preventable. For example, the Centers for Disease Control and Prevention estimates that 90% of blindness in patients with diabetes is preventable. Diabetic eye disease is the leading cause of blindness in working-age adults, and yes, 90% of this is preventable. The key to preventing blindness in this group is not by implementing some high-tech, mass screening program with costly devices. It begins with a primary care provider asking, "How is your vision for reading and driving?" and "When was your last dilated eye exam?"

In addition to describing the most common eye diseases, the authors demonstrate how important clues to ocular and systemic disease can be detected in the medical office by simple, direct observation and the use of a penlight. They describe the impact ocular disease has on things such as patient mobility, length of hospital stays for nonocular disease, hip fractures, dementia, and depression.

Our goal of this series is to convey the message that eye care and prevention of blindness begins in the primary care office with simple questions to ask your patients and tools that you use every day. Yes, we demystify the ophthalmic language, conditions, examination instruments, and laser treatments that eye care providers use. More

Med Clin N Am 105 (2021) xvii–xviii
https://doi.org/10.1016/j.mcna.2021.03.002
0025-7125/21/© 2021 Published by Elsevier Inc.

importantly, however, we impress upon this audience the fact that while the majority of vision impairment is preventable, it can only be prevented with a collaborative approach with internists, medical subspecialists, ophthalmologists, and our patients.

Paul J. Bryar, MD
Department of Ophthalmology
Northwestern University Feinberg School of Medicine
645 North Michigan Avenue
Suite 440
Chicago, IL 60611, USA

Nicholas J. Volpe, MD
Department of Ophthalmology
Northwestern University Feinberg School of Medicine
645 North Michigan Avenue
Suite 440
Chicago, IL 60611, USA

*E-mail addresses:*
p-bryar@northwestern.edu (P.J. Bryar)
nvolpe@nm.org (N.J. Volpe)

# Eye Disease in Medical Practice
## What You Should Know and Why You Should Know It

Carol H. Schmidt, MD[a,*], Nicholas J. Volpe, MD[b], Paul J. Bryar, MD[a]

**KEYWORDS**

- Eye disease • Medical practice • Vision Screening • Vision loss

**KEY POINTS**

- Incidence of cataract, diabetic retinopathy, macular degeneration, and glaucoma will significantly increase by 2050.
- Visual impairment can increase morbidity and mortality in nonocular disease.
- There are different patterns of vision loss in cataract, diabetic retinopathy, age-related macular degeneration, and glaucoma.
- Internists and medical subspecialists play an important role in prevention, detection, and early treatment of eye disease.
- Awareness of screening guidelines for eye disease as well as a basic ocular history and simple penlight examination can decrease incidence of vision loss and its impact.
- Visual impairment places a significant financial burden on society.

*The doctor of the future will give no medicines, but will interest his patients in the care of the human frame, in diet, and in the causes and prevention of disease.[1]*
*—Thomas Edison*

## INTRODUCTION

Physicians passionately pursue the prevention and treatment of disease in their patients. They cultivate productive habits, combat pain, discourage dangerous activities, provide empathy, and initiate medical and surgical treatments when indicated. In this series of vision articles, the reader will learn the vast array of visual disorders along with their impact on both individuals and society. The articles also

Conflicts of interest: The authors have no commercial or financial conflicts of interest.
[a] Northwestern University Feinberg School of Medicine, 645 North Michigan Avenue Suite 440, Chicago, IL 60611, USA; [b] Department of Ophthalmology, Northwestern University Feinberg School of Medicine, 645 North Michigan Avenue Suite 440, Chicago, IL 60611, USA
* Corresponding author.
E-mail address: c-schmidt2@northwestern.edu

Med Clin N Am 105 (2021) 397–407
https://doi.org/10.1016/j.mcna.2021.02.001
0025-7125/21/© 2021 Elsevier Inc. All rights reserved.

medical.theclinics.com

detail how visual impairment (VI) can be prevented in most patients with early detection and treatment.

Ophthalmologists devote most of their time confronting the so-called big 4 eye diseases: cataract, diabetic retinopathy, age-related macular degeneration (ARMD), and glaucoma. Prevention, diet, early detection, and medical or surgical intervention play a role in each of these diseases.[2] With regard to prevention, smoking cessation can reduce the risk of vision loss from macular degeneration. Glycemic control dramatically decreases the incidence of diabetic retinopathy. Dietary modification and specific vitamin supplements can decrease the rate of progression of macular degeneration. Identifying and early screening of those at risk for glaucoma can significantly decrease rates of glaucomatous vision loss. In addition, advances in medical and surgical treatment of these diseases have led to improved visual outcomes.

This article informs primary care providers (PCPs) and medical subspecialists on the importance of patients' visual health. It shares information on the prevalence of eye disease globally and in the United States. It addresses the costs to society and morbidity of VI. It emphasizes the profound role medical providers have in prevention and early detection of blinding conditions in their patient populations. It discusses eye diagnoses readily made in the primary care office to avoid emergency room expenses. Lastly, it reviews ophthalmic manifestations of systemic diseases.

## PREVALENCE OF VISUAL IMPAIRMENT AND EYE DISEASE

In the United States, the aging population contributes to the predicted increase in both VI and blindness, with a doubling of both parameters expected between 2015 and 2050. Six population-based studies used in the 2016 analysis by Varma and colleagues[3] included the Beaver Dam Eye Study (non-Hispanic white populations), Baltimore Eye Survey and Salisbury Eye Evaluation Study (white and African American), Proyecto VER and Los Angeles Latino eye Study (LALES; Latino/Hispanic populations), and Chinese American Eye Study (CHES; Asian American) to describe the growing scope of visual disability. The number of people with VI in the United States was estimated to be 3.22 million in 2015, and is expected to increase to 4.79 million in 2030, and to 6.95 million in 2050.[3]

With regard to prevalence and estimated increases in the big 4 eye diseases that were mentioned earlier (cataract, diabetic retinopathy, glaucoma, and macular degeneration), it is clear that health providers will encounter ever-surging numbers of patients with potentially disabling conditions. In all 4 disorders, public health specialists anticipate a doubling of affected individuals[4] (**Table 1**). Certain ethnicities will be affected to a greater extent compared with the general population. For example, Hispanic people are predicted to have a 6-fold increase in ARMD, a disease often mistakenly assumed to afflict primarily white people. The investigators report a 3-fold increase in Hispanic people with diabetic retinopathy.[5]

## COST OF VISUAL IMPAIRMENT IN THE UNITED STATES

The National Opinion Research Center Research Center (NORC) reported the cost of eye disorders and vision loss in the United States in 2013 as $139 billion, with $65

| Table 1 | | | |
|---|---|---|---|
| Prevalence projections of the big 4 visual disorders | | | |
| Condition | Individuals (Millions) 2010 | Individuals 2050 | Increase (%) |
| Cataract | 24.4 | 50 | 105 |
| Diabetic retinopathy | 7.7 | 14.6 | 89 |
| Glaucoma | 2.7 | 6.3 | 133 |
| Macular degeneration | 2.1 | 5.4 | 157 |

billion in direct medical costs. Employed individuals lost $48 billion in productivity because of VI. Long-term care of patients with VI accounts for $20 billion.[6] What is the scope of $1 billion? Spending at a rate of $1 million per month, it would take 83 years to spend a billion dollars, and, therefore, 11,537 years to spend $139 billion.

A recent analysis of Medicare data from April 2015 to 2018, by Morse and colleagues,[7] matched about 6165 individuals with normal vision to 6056 with vision loss, revealing that the latter had a 22% readmission rate, 12% higher costs, and a 4% longer hospital stay compared with controls. Similar findings were discovered in commercial health insurance patients. National extrapolation shows $500 million in additional costs for the severe VI group annually.[7]

## VISUAL IMPAIRMENT: SEEING THROUGH PATIENTS' EYES

Although escalating numbers raise alarm, medical providers consider the implications of these statistics. What does it mean for patients when clinicians say that the big 4 are increasing? The Social Security Administration defines blindness as vision less than 20/200 in the better eye or blindness as a visual field of less than 20° in the better eye for at least 12 months. The implication for patients is that they cannot drive to their appointments or read medication labels. Subtle, as well as not so subtle, disruptions of activities of daily independent living occur with VI. Patients must self-advocate and call attention to the problems. They need to find means to address these deficits; however, they often suffer silently.

Each of the diseases mentioned earlier has a different type of vision loss and vision impairment. Cataracts can cause a generalized blurring of vision with or without glare, glaucoma typically begins with peripheral vision loss, macular degeneration affects

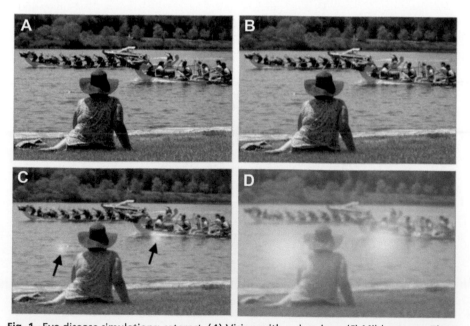

**Fig. 1.** Eye disease simulations: cataract. (*A*) Vision with a clear lens. (*B*) Mild cataract. There is a generalized mild blurriness, often described as seeing through a film. There are various types of cataract, but one of the most common is the age-related nuclear cataract, which typically slowly causes blurred vision over a period of many years. (*C*) Moderate cataract. Details on faces are no longer visible and there is the beginning of glare with reflected sunlight (*arrows*). At night, halos around light may develop. (*D*) Severe cataract. Diffuse blurred vision with glare obscuring people and objects.

the central vision, and diabetic retinopathy can cause various different patterns of vision loss. **Figs. 1–4** are simulations of what patients with vision loss can experience in these different diseases.

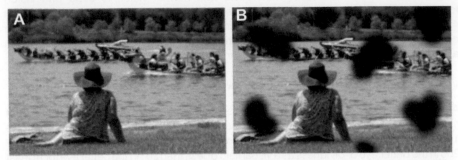

**Fig. 2.** Eye disease simulation: diabetic retinopathy. (*A*) Normal vision with no retinal disease. (*B*) Diabetic retinopathy simulation. Diabetic eye disease can be asymptomatic or have several patterns of vision loss; for example, patchy vision loss caused by intraretinal hemorrhage, central vision loss caused by macular edema, or sudden diffuse loss caused by vitreous hemorrhage. This photograph simulates patchy vision loss caused by types of diabetic eye retinopathy, including retinal hemorrhage or ischemia.

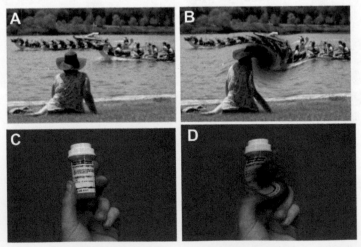

**Fig. 3.** Eye disease simulation: macular degeneration. (*A*) Normal distance vision. (*B*) Macular degeneration: distance vision simulation with loss of central vision and central distortion. (*C*) Normal near vision. (*D*) Macular degeneration: near-vision simulation with loss of central vision and distortions affecting reading. These distortions may be gradual or have abrupt onset.

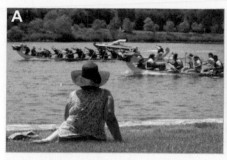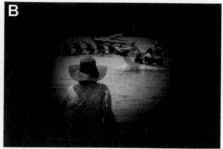

**Fig. 4.** Eye disease simulation: glaucoma. (*A*) Normal distance vision. (*B*) Glaucoma can cause various types of vision loss, but it typically involves the painless, progressive, irreversible loss of peripheral vision simulated here, which, if left untreated, will also progress to central vision loss. The most common type of glaucoma is open angle glaucoma. It is sometimes referred to as the silent thief of sight because many patients do not notice any symptoms until late in the disease course.

## VISUAL IMPAIRMENT AND RISKS TO PATIENTS' QUALITY OF LIFE AND NONOCULAR DISEASE

It is not surprising that vison loss contributes to undesirable health outcomes. Several observational studies and health surveys reach this conclusion. Medicare database analysis from 2014 done by Hamedani and colleagues[8] showed that, after adjustment for relevant comorbidities, VI is associated with hip fracture (adjusted odds ratio [AOR], 2.54), depression (AOR 3.99), anxiety (AOR 2.93), and dementia (AOR 3.91). Other investigators have provided further evidence of the relationship between VI and psychiatric/neurologic compromise. Using a powerful longitudinal study format of a Korean national sample with 1,025,340 subjects, published by a group from Hallym University College of Medicine, both the low-vision and blind subgroups had increased risk of depression. These results held after adjustment for age, sex, income, geographic factors, hypertension, diabetes, and dyslipidemia.[9] Cross-sectional analysis of 2 large datasets, the National Health and Nutrition Examination Survey (NHANES, 1999–2002) and the National Health and Aging Trends Study (NHATA 2011–2015), found decreased cognition testing parameters in study patients with low vision controlling for demographics, socioeconomic status, education level, household income, general health conditions, hearing impairment, and physical limitations.[10] VI brings risk to patients on several fronts. The effects of prevention and early detection of eye disease, as shown by the studies discussed earlier, affects the severity of nonocular diseases as well.

## ROLE OF INTERNISTS AND MEDICAL SUBSPECIALISTS IN PREVENTION OF VISUAL IMPAIRMENT AND BLINDNESS

Despite the fact that VI reduces quality of life and affects nonocular disease, providers are encouraged to know that vision loss is preventable in most patients. PCPs and medical subspecialists play a vital role in prevention of vision loss. In the case of diabetic eye disease, for example, the Diabetes Control and Complications Trial (DCCT) concluded that, in type 1 diabetes, a 10% reduction in hemoglobin $A_{1c}$ level (eg, from 10% to 9% or from 8% to 7.2%) reduced the risk of retinopathy progression by 43%.[11] Greater than 70% of respondents in the National Eye Health Education Program (NEHEP) 2005 Public Knowledge, Attitudes, and Practices Survey thought that loss of their eyesight would have the greatest impact on daily life; however, less than 11% knew that early diabetic retinopathy and glaucoma lacked symptoms.[12] Providers can channel patients' concern for loss of vision into productive conversations to motivate patients in a range of areas, including glycemic control, smoking cessation, healthy diet, medication compliance, and screening guideline compliance. Patients benefit when their providers gather relevant ocular history, use simple examination techniques such as direct observation or penlight examination, and include appropriate eye-screening recommendations into patients' care plans.

Here are some simple steps that internists or medical subspecialists can incorporate into their daily practice that can dramatically decrease vision loss and its impact on their patients.

## History

Ask appropriate visually-directed questions. The question, "Can you see well?" will not bring out the same information as, "Are you struggling with small print or seeing road signs at night?" Take interest in eye-drop instructions and eye vitamins on patient medication lists. PCPs are frequently asked by patients to fill glaucoma drops along with other systemic medications with 90 day/3 refills. Knowledge that a typical patient with glaucoma is seen 2 to 4 times per year by an ophthalmologist should prompt PCPs to inquire when the patient last presented to an eye doctor. This conversation identifies patients with glaucoma who repeatedly request their PCPs refill their drops, and are lost to follow-up, while glaucoma, the silent thief of sight, causes further irreversible vision loss.

PCPs often ask patients about risk prevention, such as wearing seatbelts or a bicycle helmet. If a patient's profession is high risk for eye trauma, ask whether the patient routinely wears safety glasses. The National Institute for Occupational Safety and Health (NIOSH) reports that every day about 2000 US workers sustain job-related eye injuries that require medical treatment. Safety experts and eye doctors believe proper eye protection lessens the severity or prevents 90% of these eye injuries.[13]

## Examination

PCPs can detect eye disease or ocular manifestations of systemic disease without fancy slit lamps and cumbersome direct ophthalmoscopes. Careful direct observation (droopy eyelid, red eye, exophthalmos, and so forth) can detect many conditions **(Table 2)**.

**Table 2**
**Examples of ocular diseases that can be diagnosed by penlight examination**

| Observation | Condition Suspected |
| --- | --- |
| Corneal arcus in patients <50 y old or with xanthelasma | Hypercholesterolemia |
| White corneal opacity with red eye | Corneal ulcer |
| Loss of iris detail | Hyphema |
| Exophthalmos | Thyroid-related eye disease |
| Prominent diffuse eye vascularization | Cavernous-carotid fistula |
| Anisocoria | Subarachnoid hemorrhage |
| Restricted eye movement | Vascular muscle palsy, thyroid-related eye disease, myasthenia gravis |
| Eyelid mass with loss of eyelashes | Basal, squamous, or sebaceous cell carcinoma |

Is there a focal white spot on the cornea in a contact lens wearer that is consistent with a corneal ulcer? Is there limited view to see the iris in a patient who took a tennis ball to the face? Lack of iris detail suggests blood in the front of the eye, called hyphema, with potential associated conditions such as increased eye pressure. Does the provider notice a restriction of eye movement in gaze positions in a vasculopathic patient with new-onset double vision?

An observation of a white ring in the peripheral cornea can be extremely important (**Fig. 5**). This ring is called corneal arcus. It is very common in patients more than 65 years of age and is typically not associated with any other systemic disease. However, if this is seen in patients younger than 55 years, this can be the only sign on physical examination of a patient with hyperlipidemia.

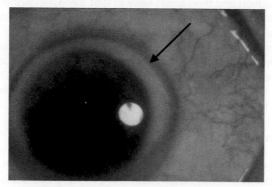

**Fig. 5.** Corneal arcus is a white ring in the peripheral cornea (*arrow*). This ring can be seen in younger patients with hyperlipidemia, or more commonly in patients older than 65 years. Used with permission, © 2021 American Academy of Ophthalmology.

Without regularly performing direct ophthalmoscopy, it is unlikely that a non–eye care provider will develop sufficient skill to make meaningful observations. In our opinion, it is much more valuable for PCPs to remind patients about the importance of regular screening eye examinations by an eye care provider. Nonmydriatic fundus cameras are becoming increasingly available and affordable. They may become ubiquitous in primary care or medical subspecialty offices in the near future. These cameras, combined with cloud-based or artificial intelligence–based services to review and read images, may soon greatly enhance successful eye disease screening.

A surprising number of eye problems find their way directly to the emergency department (ED). Many PCPs can easily triage with penlight and treat in the standard office. In a study of 12 million ED visits for ocular issues from 2006 to 2011, 44% were considered nonemergent. Of these, 4 million visits were for conjunctivitis, subconjunctival hemorrhage in the absence of trauma, and styes. Forty-one percent of the ED visits in the study were classified as emergent, and included corneal abrasion and foreign body.[14]

## Follow-up Care Plan: Ocular Screening Examinations and Risk Assessment

### Screening eye examinations

In the absence of eye disease or systemic disease requiring eye screening, the American Academy of Ophthalmology (AAO) 2016 Preferred Practice Patterns recommends comprehensive eye examinations for patients without risk factors or other ocular disease based on age.[15] Recommendations on the frequency of dilated eye examinations for patients with no eye disease or need for corrective lenses vary by age. People less than 40 years old should have one every 5 to 10 years, between 40 and 54 years old every 2 to 4 years, 55 to 64 years old every 1 to 3 years, and annually for those 65 years of age and older. Although optometrists and ophthalmologists are capable of performing screening or surveillance eye examinations, as medical doctors, ophthalmologists have greater familiarity with systemic diseases and are equipped to provide necessary medical and surgical treatments.

Patients with diabetes require eye screening based on the type and duration of their disease. Type 1 patients need examinations within 5 years of diagnosis and yearly thereafter. Type 2 patients need referral at the time of initial diagnosis and yearly thereafter. Some guidelines allow for a diabetic eye examination every 2 years if the prior examination was normal.[16] Pregnant women with type 1 or 2 diabetes need examinations before conception and then again early in first trimester. Adherence to diabetic eye screening is arguably the most effective way to prevent VI and blindness in adults less than 65 years of age.

Patients who are at risk of other eye diseases (eg, African Americans and Hispanic people for glaucoma or patients with a strong family history of glaucoma) may need more frequent screening, perhaps every 1 to 2 years for those age 40 years and older.

Patients taking certain medications, such as hydroxychloroquine or ethambutol, require screening for ocular toxicity.

### Smoking cessation

A repetitious and multifaceted approach is often necessary to convince patients to quit smoking. Smoking cessation decreases the incidence of cardiovascular disease and cancer in addition to many other diseases, including eye disease. Nonsmokers decrease their risk of vision loss and blindness associated with macular degeneration and glaucoma. Armed with this information, medical providers have another approach to discussing smoking cessation with their patients.

### Driving

PCPs must consider several criteria in their discussions about driving privileges with concerned patients and their families. PCPs realize that driving safety and patient well-being are more than seatbelt use. Older patients carry higher risk of serious injury in even minor car accidents with air bag deployment. However, loss of driving privileges can dramatically affect independence in some patients. Some of the driving criteria are objective. These criteria include the presence of medical conditions (frequent seizures) or use of medications contraindicated with driving. Other parameters are more difficult to quantify, such as declining cognitive or motor skills. Knowledge of the state's vision requirements and the role of the PCP in the conversation helps wise decisions to be made.

Visual requirements vary state by state, with most states requiring the best-corrected vision to be 20/40 or better in 1 eye for night driving. In some states, the threshold is not as stringent. The best-corrected vision can be 20/70 or better if other criteria are met, such as the worse eye being better than 20/200. Some states have a minimum peripheral visual field requirement, whereas others do not. If a patient fails the state's vision screen in the licensure process, then most states refer that patient for a formal eye examination. The eye doctor provides specific information, such as uncorrected and best-corrected visual acuity, peripheral vision measurements, and ocular condition stability. Fortunately, the results of the eye examination are reported as either pass or fail. Meeting the vision requirements does not necessarily indicate that the patient should drive, but failure to meet the standards may help the patient accept the decision not to drive. Failure on the vision component may assist the primary provider when resentful patients disagree over equivocal cognitive and motor skill evaluations.

## PRESENTING SIGNS/SYMPTOMS OF SYSTEMIC DISEASE WITH OCULAR FINDINGS

Ocular disorders accompany systemic diseases. The AAO published a useful guide in 2009 on the topic of ocular manifestations of systemic disease, which the authors encourage readers to review.[17] The fascinating scope of this topic is beyond the limits

**Table 3**
**Systemic disease with eye manifestations**

| Category | Example of Condition | Systemic Signs/ Symptoms | Ocular Signs/Symptoms |
|---|---|---|---|
| Congenital | Neurofibromatosis | Skin macules | Iris lesions (Lisch nodules), optic nerve glioma |
| | Marfan syndrome | Cardiac disease | High refractive error, dislocated lens |
| Traumatic | Shaken baby syndrome | Multiple fractures in different stages of healing | Vitreous, preretinal, intraretinal hemorrhage |
| Vascular | Embolic disease | Carotid bruit, heart murmur | Retina emboli (Hollenhorst plaque), painless monocular vision loss |
| | Hyperviscosity syndrome | Abnormal complete blood count parameters | Intraretinal hemorrhages, optic disc congestion |
| Neoplastic | Metastatic carcinoma | Mammogram/ computed tomography abnormality based on primary source | Choroidal masses with or without vision loss |
| Autoimmune | Collagen vascular disorders | Laboratory antibody abnormalities | Dry eye, uveitis, corneal melts |
| | System lupus erythematous | Neurologic, kidney, cardiac malfunctions | Above findings, plus retinal vasculitis |
| | Sarcoidosis | Multisystem computed tomography chest lymphadenopathy | Uveitis, lacrimal gland enlargement, optic disc infiltration |
| Idiopathic | Intracranial hypertension | Headache | Papilledema, visual field defects |
| | Multiple sclerosis | MRI abnormalities | Painful vison loss |
| Infectious | Acquired immunodeficiency syndrome | Laboratory value abnormalities, CD4, and so forth Pneumonia | Red conjunctival mass (Kaposi sarcoma), Retina disorder: cotton wool spots, retinitis with hemorrhagic white necrotic patches |

of this article, but a representative sample of ocular findings in certain systemic diseases is presented (**Table 3**).

## SUMMARY

Eye disease and vision impairment have a significant impact on patients and society. In addition to the limitations in vision, VI negatively affects morbidity and mortality of nonocular disease. Internists and medical subspecialists play a vital role in the prevention, detection, and treatment of eye disease, which adds significantly to patients' quality of life. Primary providers are called on to take ocular history, perform penlight examinations, recognize screening guidelines, and to incorporate these elements into patient care plans. Most VI is preventable, and a collaborative approach with patients, internists, medical subspecialists, and eye care providers is essential in preserving vision.

## CLINICS CARE POINTS

- Glycemic control reduces the risk of visual impairment in patients with insulin dependent diabetes such that a 10% deduction in HgA1C reduces risk of retinopathy progression by 43%.

- Type 1 diabetics should have dilated eye exams within 5 years of diagnosis and yearly thereafter. Type 2 diabetics need referral for fundus exam at diagnosis and yearly thereafter.

- Smoking cessation reduces the risk of vision loss from macular degeneration.

- Visual impairment erodes quality of life with increased morbidity and mortality in association with non-ocular diseases.

- Asking visually-directed questions regarding activities of daily living such as the utilization protective eyewear for those with high-risk professions or hobbies improve outcomes for our patients.

- Current recommendations for eye exams for patients without eye disease are every 1-3 years for ages 55-64 and annually for patients over 65.

## ACKNOWLEDGMENTS

The authors would like to acknowledge Kaitlyn Veto for the photographs in **Figs. 1–4**. This work was supported by an unrestricted departmental grant from Research to Prevent Blindness.

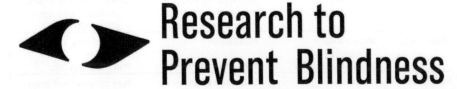

## REFERENCES

1. Available at: http://www.goodreads.com/quotes/13639-the-doctor-of-the-futre-will-give-no-medication-but. Accessed September 19, 2020.

2. Glaucoma Research Foundation. Available at: http://www.glaucoma.org/treatment/what-vitamins-and-nutrients-will-help-prevent-my-glaucoma-from-worsening.php. Accessed December 28,2020.

3. Varma R, Vajaranaut TS, Burkemper B, et al. Visual Impairment and Blindness in Adults in the United States. JAMA Ophthalmol 2016;134(7):802–9.

4. National Eye Institute. Eye Health Data and Statistics. Available at: https://www.nei.nih.gov/learn-about-eye-health/resources-for-health-educators/eye-health-data-and-statistics/cataract-data-and-statistics   https://www.nei.nih.gov/learn-about-eye-health/resources-for-health-educators/eye-health-data-and-statistics/diabetic-retinopathy-data-and-statistics  https://www.nei.nih.gov/learn-about-eye-health/resources-for-health-educators/eye-health-data-and-statistics/glaucoma-data-and-statistics  https://www.nei.nih.gov/learn-about-eye-health/resources-for-health-educators/eye-health-data-and-statistics/age-related-macular-degeneration-amd-data-and-statistics. Accessed January 2, 2021.

5. Wittenborn JS, Rein DB. The future of vision: Forecasting the prevalence and cost of vison problems. Chicago: NORC at the University of Chicago Prepared for Prevent Blindness; 2014.

6. Available at: https://www.norc.org/Research/Projects/Pages/the-economic-burden-of-vision-loss-and-eye-disorders-in-the-united-states.aspx#:-:text   Accessed September 13, 2020.

7. Morse AR, Seiple W, Talwar N, et al. MS association of vison loss with hospital use and costs among older adults. JAMA Ophthalmol 2019;137(6):634–40.

8. Hamedani AG, VanderBeek BL, Willis AL. Ophthalmic Blindness and VI in the Medicare population: disparities and association with hip fracture and neuropsychiatric outcome. Ophthalmic Epidemiol 2019;26(4):279–85.

9. Choi HG, Lee MJ, Lee SM. Visual impairment and risk of depression. A longitudinal follow-up study using a national sample cohort. Sci Rep 2018;8:2083.

10. Chen SP, Bhattacharaya J, Pershing MD. Association of Vision Loss with Cognition in Older Adults. JAMA Ophthalmol 2017;135(9):963–70.

11. The Diabetes Control and Complications Trial Research Group. The relationship of glycemic exposure (HbA$_{1c}$) to the risk of development and progression of retinopathy in the Diabetes Control and Complications Trial. Diabetes 1995;44:968–83.

12. Centers for Disease Control. Available at: https://www.cdc.gov/visionhealth/basics/ced/fastfacts.htm. Accessed September 19, 2020.

13. Centers for Disease Control. Available at: https://www.cdc.gov/niosh/topics/eye/. Accessed September 19, 2020.

14. Roomasa C, Zafar SY, Canner JK, et al. Epidemiology of Eye-Related Emergency Department Visits. Ophthalmology 2016;134(4):312–9.

15. Stephen M, Feder RS. 2016 AAO preferred practice patterns. Elsevier; 2015.

16. Solomon SD, Chew E, Duh EJ, et al. Diabetic Retinopathy: A Position Statement by the American Diabetes Association. Diabetes Care 2017;40(3):412–8.

17. 2009 AAO Ocular Manifestations of Systemic Disease Speaker Notes. Karla J. Johns, MD Executive Editor. Rosa A. Tang, MD with Ophthalmology Liaisons Committee of the AAO. Eye Care Skills: Presentations for Physicians and Other Health Care Professionals Version 3.0. Available at: http://www.med.virginia.edu/ophthalmology/wp-content/uploads/sites/295/2015/12/Systemic.pdf.   Accessed December 28, 2020.

# Ocular Complaints, Disease, and Emergencies in the General Medical Setting

Cynthia A. Bradford, MD*, Andrew T. Melson, MD

## KEYWORDS

- Ocular complaints • Red eye • Vision loss • Double vision

## KEY POINTS

- Primary care providers must rely on an accurate and thorough history to differentiate ocular disease. History alone can dictate the need for urgent or emergent referral.
- Red eyes are commonly due to viral conjunctivitis, but red flags include persistent refractory disease, copious purulent discharge, periocular dermatologic changes, or recent ocular trauma.
- Acute vision loss should prompt urgent evaluation, and in elderly patients, giant cell arteritis must be considered.
- Double vision is more likely neurologic when it goes away with monocular occlusion or is worse when looking in certain directions of gaze.
- Primary care physicians play an essential role in ensuring appropriate ophthalmic screening for diabetes, glaucoma, and medication toxicity.

## INTRODUCTION

Primary care physicians constitute about one-third of US physicians but perform about one-half of all clinical visits.[1] It is natural that patients share concerns regarding their eyes with their primary physician. Loss of vision is a common fear, particularly in elderly patients. Loss of independence with driving and being able to perform tasks such as reading and paying bills drastically affects quality of life and can lead to depression. A study found that about 2% to 3% of all primary care patient visits involve ocular complaints.[2] The presenting conditions consisted of the following general categories: minor inflammatory, traumatic conditions and foreign bodies, visual disturbances, and eyelid problems. The 2 most common problems presenting to primary care physicians were conjunctivitis and corneal abrasion.

Department of Ophthalmology, University of Oklahoma, College of Medicine, Dean A. McGee Eye Institute, 608 Stanton L. Young Boulevard, Oklahoma City, OK 73104, USA
* Corresponding author.
*E-mail address:* Cynthia-bradford@dmei.org

Med Clin N Am 105 (2021) 409–423
https://doi.org/10.1016/j.mcna.2021.02.002
0025-7125/21/© 2021 Elsevier Inc. All rights reserved.

medical.theclinics.com

## OCULAR PRESENTING COMPLAINTS

As with other organ systems, an accurate and complete history is key to making the correct diagnosis in patients with ocular complaints. Many patients refer to their complaints in vague or anatomically inaccurate terms that can lead one down a false pathway. Patients will often talk about "their eye" when they are really talking about their eyelid or periocular structures. Another common confusion with history taking is when a patient describes "something in their eye," do they mean something they see when looking out or something they see when looking at their eye in a mirror? When taking a history of visual complaints, always clarify the circumstances under which complaints occur. If a patient describes double vision, always ask if it is at near, at distance, only in certain directions of gaze, and with their distance glasses on or off. Patients who wear glasses to see in the distance may notice double vision at a distance without their glasses!

Whether the complaint is about vision, redness, or pain, the points to clarify are similar to historical elements of complaints about other parts of the body. It is important to know if the problem is noticed in one or both eyes. Ocular diseases due to underlying systemic disease or age-related degenerated processes often affect both eyes, although they may be asymmetric in presentation. On the other hand, infectious processes or vascular occlusions typically present with only unilateral involvement at least in the early stages.

If the complaint is vision loss, the temporal profile of loss can help identify the diagnosis. Was the vision loss slow and progressive over months or was it sudden, complete vision loss? Is the visual loss central or is it peripheral? Patients can often describe the visual field loss such as top or bottom part of vision missing or just a superior or inferior quadrant missing. Inferior loss is noticed more often due to looking down while working or walking. Similarly, the temporal field of view is larger and patients with a homonymous hemianopia will often complain about temporal field loss in one eye but may fail to recognize the nasal field loss in their contralateral eye.

A visual complaint of double vision could be due to ocular motility or alignment problem. The most important differentiating factor is whether the double vision remains present when covering either eye. True binocular diplopia is only present when both eyes are open. The patient should be able to answer if the images are side by side or one on top of the other. Although monocular double vision is rarely urgent, double vision that is worse in a specific direction of gaze is more likely to be neurologic in cause.

Patients will often describe features diagnostic for their condition if you listen closely. For example, a patient may say the only problem is when they bend over, they go completely blind, but the vision returns after a few seconds once they stand up. This is called transient visual obscuration and is a temporary, reversible cause of positional vision loss in patients with papilledema, often from idiopathic intracranial hypertension. These subtle differentiations in symptomatology are essential to primary care providers who otherwise may have limited examination findings to hone in on a diagnosis.

### *Vision*

#### *Common problems*
#### Not vision threatening

   **Dry eyes** The cause of dry eyes is multifactorial and becomes more common with increasing age. Patients often complain of an intermittent blur that clears with blinking or use of lubricant drops. Symptoms increase with extended computer use, reading, driving, or any intense visual task that reduces blinking frequency.

Patients with dry eyes may describe quick, sharp pains or a sandy, gritty sensation. Some patients complain predominately of intermittent tearing, whereas others complain of ocular discharge. The discharge can be confused with infection, but it is excess mucous production secondary to dryness. Lubricant drops can be used to rinse mucus out. It is important that the patient does not pick at the eye to retrieve the mucus, as this can cause recurrent microtrauma that exacerbates the condition.

Initial treatment of dry eyes is with over-the-counter lubricant eye drops. Many patients will turn to allergy drops or ones that "get the red out," but these contain vaso-constricting agents that are counterproductive to long-term ocular surface health. Allergies can exacerbate dryness, but the predominate symptom is usually itching. At a minimum, lubricant drops should be used first thing in the morning and before bedtime. Most over-the-counter lubricant drops contain preservatives and should not be used in excess of 3 to 4 times a day. Preservative-free lubricant eye drops are available, which can be used more frequently if necessary. Gel drops are a thicker formulation that coat the ocular surface for a longer period of time. Patients will need to try different types of drops sequentially to learn which one works best for them. Drop use is more effective when used routinely for preventative maintenance rather than as needed when the eyes feel dry.

In addition to ocular lubrication, warm compresses (with a damp warm wash cloth over the closed eyelids for 3–5 minutes) at bedtime can help to reduce symptoms by allowing the meibomian glands to function more effectively. Oral doxycycline, 50 to 100 mg/d, can also be used for symptomatic relief of inflammatory dry eye, particularly in those with ocular rosacea. Both of these treatments may take months to achieve maximum effectiveness. More advanced dry eye treatments including prescription drops and procedural interventions are available through eye care specialists.

There are a variety of systemic diseases that have increased incidence of dry eye. Immune-mediated disorders such as Sjögren syndrome, rheumatoid arthritis, systemic lupus erythematosus, and graft-versus-host, among others, have strong associations with ocular surface disease. Other disorders such Parkinson's, Bell's palsy, and thyroid eye disease are also associated with dry eye disease due to decreased blink and increased exposure. Many oral medications, including antihistamines, certain antidepressants, and some hormone replacement medications, may cause or worsen dry eye. Environmental factors can exacerbate dryness, including low humidity, wind, and ceiling fans that desiccate the ocular surface.

**Floaters** The vitreous jelly is a solid gel at birth that is firmly adherent to the retina and optic nerve. Over a lifetime, the gel becomes liquified and develops floating fibers. There comes a time in all patients, earlier in those with myopia, when the vitreous attachment to the optic nerve starts to pull away. This typically occurs between the ages of 45 and 65 years. The result is the sudden onset of visually bothersome floaters, sometimes accompanied with perception of brief flashes of light most noticeable in the dark. This is called a posterior vitreous detachment (PVD). These common, but annoying, floaters are more often noticed in high relief, for example, when looking at the blue sky, a bland wall, or a computer screen. The floaters are generally described as stringy and may have veil-like movement across the field of vision, even when the eye is held still. Sudden PVD is a risk factor for the creation of a retinal tear, which has similar symptoms but requires urgent treatment.[3] Patients with sudden onset of new floaters should be referred to an ophthalmologist for further evaluation, as historical elements alone cannot determine the diagnosis (**Fig. 1**).

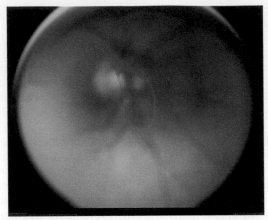

**Fig. 1.** Posterior vitreous detachment (PVD) is a partial or complete separation of the posterior vitreous cortex from the internal limiting membrane of the retina. (This image was originally published in the Retina Image Bank® website. Alex P. Hunyor MD. Posterior vitreous detachment. Retina Image Bank. 2013; # 3073. © the American Society of Retina Specialists".)

### Vision threatening

**Distorted central vision** Central visual distortion is an indication of irregularity in the central retina (an area known as the macula). Many patients will describe that an object that they know to be vertical (door jamb for instance) seems crooked or wavy. Most often, these symptoms of metamorphopsia are due to a wrinkle in the retina, exudative (wet) age-related macular degeneration, or other less common retinal problems. Hearing a patient complain of central wavy distortion to their vision should prompt referral to comprehensive ophthalmologist or retinal specialist, if available (**Fig. 2**).

**Peripheral vision loss** Peripheral vision loss is less specific and can be due to neurologic or ocular causes. Cortical causes of vision loss affect BOTH eyes in all

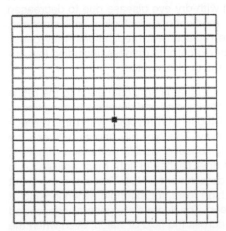 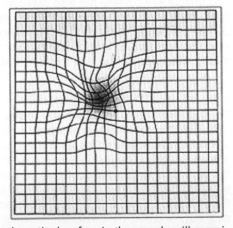

**Fig. 2.** Distortion. Patients with irregularity in the retinal surface in the macula will experience metamorphopsia, which is distortion in their vision. They will describe that fences are not straight or the door jamb bows. When shown an Amsler grid, which highlights distortion, they will not see straight lines, but distorted, as shown in the second picture. (*Courtesy*: National Eye Institute, National Institutes of Health (NEI/NIH)).

circumstances, and the associated visual field defects will respect the vertical midline of the field of vision in each eye. Strokes or tumors of the cortical visual pathways result in homonymous field defects, affecting the left or right side of vision in each eye. Patients may only recognize the field loss in their temporal field of view, so confrontation visual field testing of each eye individually must be performed to identify homonymous field defects. Similarly, parasellar masses can lead to temporal field changes in both eyes that respect the vertical midline and lead to symmetric tunneling of vision.

Ocular causes of peripheral field loss do not routinely respect the vertical midline and are often asymmetric between the eyes. Bilateral causes are often degenerative in nature, and a family history of glaucoma or inherited diseases of the retina may be elicited. Optic nerve–related changes often present unilaterally and can have associated color desaturation or vision loss respecting the horizontal midline. Unilateral causes of vision loss are varied and should similarly prompt referral to a specialist.

**Concerning floaters** Patients experiencing floaters from a visually threatening process will tell you that the new floaters they have are "different" from previous floaters. They will often describe hundreds of tiny black floaters that are seen at all times in one eye, "like a swarm of gnats." Possible causes are retinal tear/detachment, vitreous hemorrhage, or inflammation in the eye. With the direct ophthalmoscope, it is possible to see floating debris in red reflex. If there is a severe intraocular hemorrhage, no red reflex may be visible at all. Retinal detachment will present with a progressive visual field defect that can be mapped out with confrontational fields testing. New onset of atypical floaters in one eye requires urgent referral to comprehensive ophthalmologist or retinal specialist, if available (**Fig. 3.**)

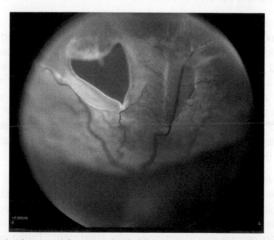

**Fig. 3.** Superior retinal tear with associated detachment. ("This image was originally published in the Retina Image Bank® website. Jason S. Calhoun MD. Horseshoe retinal tear. Retina Image Bank 2013; #7030. © the American Society of Retina Specialists.")

**Acute visual loss** Sudden, painless visual loss is an emergency and is most often an arterial occlusive event. Occlusion of the central retinal artery results in near-complete blindness and is unilateral in almost all circumstances. Branch retinal artery occlusions will have focal areas of unilateral vision loss, typically involving one quadrant of vision. Both are considered stroke equivalents and require workup to exclude embolic or systemic causes.[4] Similarly, occlusion of small vessels that supply the optic nerve can result in sudden painless vision loss known as ischemic optic neuropathy, which is typically described as a loss of the upper or lower half of field of vision and is associated with nocturnal hypotension, obstructive sleep apnea, and use of phosphodiesterase inhibitors. Ischemic optic neuropathy is an irreversible cause of vision loss and is among the feared consequences of unrecognized giant cell arteritis (GCA) (**Fig. 4**).

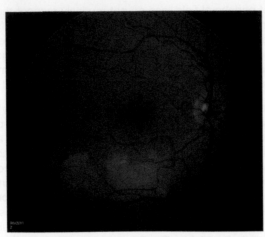

**Fig. 4.** Right eye. Inferior branch artery occlusion due to calcium emboli from cardiac valve. Whitening of the retina is the area of ischemia.

Amaurosis fugax is a *transient* monocular vision loss event caused by vascular occlusion with a gradual return of vision as the vasculature reperfuses. Although most events are related to emboli and warrant workup as such, one must not neglect to consider arteritis as a potential cause. GCA is of particular concern if the episodes are recurrent and associated with headache, scalp tenderness, or jaw claudication. Patients will often provide stunning descriptions of their vision blacking out followed by a reblooming of their vision back to normal repeatedly. These patients require immediate steroid treatment and referral for consideration of temporal artery biopsy by a trained specialist (**Fig. 5**).

**Subacute sudden vision loss** Subacute vision loss can have a wide variety of causes, most of which require specialty evaluation. Retinal vein occlusions present with more insidious loss of vision compared with their arterial counterparts. The resulting venous congestion leads to slow exudation of fluid, which reduces quality of central vision and can require long-term specialty treatment. These occlusions occur more frequently in patients with chronic microvascular risk factors such as diabetes, hypertension, and hypercholesterolemia.

Subacute vision loss associated with *pain* should raise concern for possible optic neuritis, particularly when found in combination with other neurologic complaints. Most patients with optic neuritis will describe unilateral vision loss (color desaturation initially) over the course of a few days and pain that is worse with eye movements. Unlike ocular surface discomfort that may improve with blinking, painful causes of vision loss that do not improve with simple measures require urgent evaluation.

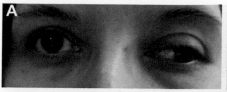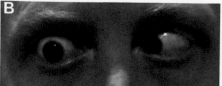

**Fig. 5.** Giant cell arteritis is a disease with potentially devastating visual consequences if unrecognized and untreated. The wide variation in clinical presentation and lack of specific biomarker requires that providers have a high index of suspicion for disease. Photo A is a patient presenting with scalp necrosis. High-dose steroid treatment is very effective but requires long-term treatment and has many adverse effects. As such, temporal artery biopsy should be performed for confirmation in all patients suspected to have the disease. Photo B shows patient prior to temporal artery biopsy.

- Common but nonspecific features:
  - Headache, scalp tenderness, fatigue, fever, weight loss
- Less common but more specific features:
  - Jaw claudication, polymyalgia rheumatica, scalp necrosis (photo), temporal artery prominence/thickening (photo)

**Double vision** The first step in evaluating double vision is always to determine if it is monocular or binocular. Monocular diplopia remains present despite occlusion of one eye and is almost never neurologic in nature. Similarly, a complaint of triple or quadruple vision is nonneurologic. True binocular diplopia can be horizontal, vertical, or oblique in nature and goes away with occlusion of either eye. There are many potential causes of acquired double vision in adulthood. Ones with insidious onset are typically decompensations of preexisting childhood strabismus, but those with acute onset require more urgent evaluation.

Certain features of double vision are red flags that can help the primary care provider identify dangerous disease processes. Specifically, any double vision associated with asymmetry of pupils or eyelid position should raise concern for a more acute cause. Pupil involving third nerve palsies MUST be rapidly imaged to rule out aneurysmal compression.[5] Other red flags include diplopia associated with any ocular motility restriction on examination. Because these red flags can be subtle, asking the patient if the double vision is worse in one direction of gaze compared with another can be very helpful in eliciting a history of worrisome incomitance. Large fluctuations in double vision or eyelid position throughout the day can help identify myasthenia gravis (**Fig. 6**).

### Red Eye

History and symptoms are the most helpful ways to separate the common causes of a red eye.

### Subconjunctival hemorrhage
Subconjunctival hemorrhage is often a source of great concern to patients but is almost always benign. They typically occur with eye rubbing, trauma, or Valsalva. If recurrent, ask about contact lens usage, check for uncontrolled blood pressure, consider hematologic disease or anticoagulant effect, and refer to further ocular evaluation, if uncertain.

### Conjunctivitis
Conjunctivitis is the most common cause of a red eye. Because of its frequency, it is often seen and treated by a primary care physician. The various types of conjunctivitis can seem similar, but history and symptoms help to differentiate the cause.

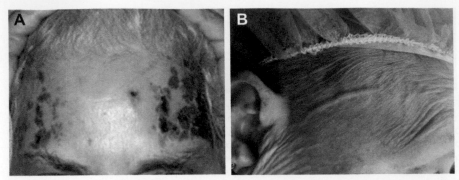

**Fig. 6.** New onset of oculomotor (third) cranial nerve palsy (photo A) requires neuroimaging. Pupil involvement raises concern for aneurysmal compression and should prompt urgent evaluation with CTA or MRA. Partial third nerve palsies may lack classic signs of marked ptosis or obvious motility deficits, and any patients with anisocoria and diplopia should be carefully evaluated. Trochlear (fourth) cranial nerve palsies will often have subtle findings of vertical diplopia worse in certain directions of gaze and are most commonly due to trauma or microvascular mononeuropathy when acquired. Abducens (sixth) nerve palsy will manifest with horizontal diplopia worse in lateral gaze with more readily identifiable abduction deficit (photo B). Referral for further evaluation is indicated, as a wide variety of potential causes exist, including elevated intracranial pressure, skull base lesions, trauma, cavernous sinus disease, and many others.

Special note: conjunctivitis associated with soft contact lens wear can be more complex. These patients should stop wearing their contacts and urgently see their contact lens provider. Decreased vision, purulent discharge, or pain should prompt referral to an ophthalmologist emergently.

### Viral conjunctivitis
Viruses are the most common cause of conjunctivitis and are often very contagious. Typically, these are due to one of several types of adenovirus and presents with a red irritated eye, watery discharge, and potentially systemic viral symptoms. In most cases, involvement of one eye is followed by second eye involvement within 24 to 48 hours. There is often a history of exposure to someone with a red eye or a small child with a viral illness. The viral particles can remain infective on hard surfaces for several weeks, and the physician should discuss the importance of hygiene to limit spread of the disease. To avoid infecting others at home and the workplace, a recommendation should be made to self-isolate for 7 to 14 days from the onset of symptoms in the second eye. Length of isolation can be discussed with the patient and may vary by job type and duration of symptoms. Most cases are mild, but some can be severe and will need to be referred to an ophthalmologist.

On examination, the eyes are injected, and there can be lid swelling. There is only watery discharge, and patient may have a preauricular node. Patients with these symptoms should not be left in waiting room but isolated in an examination room. Providers should use personal protective equipment and avoid direct skin to skin contact.[6] After the patient leaves, careful cleaning of all surfaces will help prevent infection of other patients or office staff. Outpatient offices have been the source of widespread public health outbreaks of epidemic keratoconjunctivitis due to insufficient preventative measures.[7]

There is no curative treatment of viral conjunctivitis, and support measures consist of preservative-free lubricant drops and cool compresses. Antibiotic drops are not indicated and are very painful on the inflamed conjunctiva. Just as in viral bronchitis, viral conjunctivitis can develop a secondary bacterial infection that would manifest with worsening symptoms and purulent discharge. Keeping the eye lids clean helps prevent a secondary infection. Less commonly herpes simplex, herpes zoster, or molluscum can cause conjunctivitis, illustrating the importance of a careful examination of the periocular skin.

### Bacterial conjunctivitis
The most common bacterial conjunctivitis is mild and usually self-limited. Patients often report waking up with lashes stuck together with mattering. The infection causes a grainy sensation with pain. Treatment for 5 to 7 days with inexpensive broad spectrum topical antibiotic relieves the symptoms more rapidly. Patients with recurrent episodes of mild conjunctivitis often have blepharitis, and the underlying lid disease must be treated to clear the conjunctivitis.

More aggressive bacterial conjunctivitis produces purulent discharge. Copious purulent discharge suggests gonococcal infection, and if suspected, emergent referral to an ophthalmologist is warranted. Methicillin-resistant *Staphylococcus aureus* and chlamydia are other causes of complex conjunctivitis that may fail conservative empirical treatment.

Chronic unilateral conjunctivitis can be caused by noninfectious mimickers of bacterial conjunctivitis such as neoplasia or autoimmune processes. Conjunctival lymphomas and carcinomas may be subtle in the early stages. Autoimmune causes of uveitis or scleritis can seem similar to conjunctivitis but have severe photophobia and pain in most circumstances. Patients with rosacea-associated blepharitis can have a chronic conjunctival injection and lid disease that is amenable to treatment.

### Allergic conjunctivitis
Seasonal or perennial allergic conjunctivitis is common and presents with red itchy eyes and boggy eyelid edema. Simple recommendations are to avoid the allergen and to use cool compresses and refrigerated lubricant eye drops. Bathing and washing the hair after exposure to allergen is helpful. Avoid rubbing the eyes. There are many over-the-counter drops to improve allergy symptoms, including antihistamine drops, combination antihistamine with decongestants, and combination antihistamine with mast cell stabilizers. Steroid drops should be avoided due to side effects that need to be monitored by an ophthalmologist. Some patients are relieved with simple oral antihistamines.

Vernal and atopic conjunctivitis are specific disease entities above and beyond typical allergic conjunctivitis. They tend to occur in younger individuals with other atopic symptoms and can progress to significant visual compromise. Thickened eyelid skin, photophobia, and severe recurrent seasonal disease should prompt specialty evaluation, as steroids are needed to manage these patients.

Allergic conjunctivitis can also form as a reaction to a topical drop or medication. Common culprits are aminoglycoside drops, glaucoma drops, and even the preservative used in most over-the-counter drops (benzalkonium chloride). Stopping the drops will result in improvement in a few days. Continuing the drops can lead to a contact dermatitis of the lids, with thickened, red skin. Systemic immune reactions such as Stevens-Johnson syndrome- and mycoplasma-induced rash and mucositis can present with severe conjunctivitis as well.

### Chemical conjunctivitis
Exposure of caustic chemical substances results in a red, irritated eye. The degree of involvement can span from a simple irritation that resolves in a day to severe, vision-

threatening chemical injury resulting in an ocular emergency. If a patient calls with a splash injury to eye, they should be instructed to rinse the eye with eye rinse or simple tap water for 5 minutes. If the chemical is known to be toxic to the eye, such as alkaline solutions or acidic solutions, they should proceed to nearest emergency room. Attempts at neutralization of the chemical should be avoided, as these reactions are exothermic and can worsen ocular damage.

## Ocular Pain

### Without trauma

Mild pain is frequently due to dryness and is accompanied by a sensation of scratchiness or sand in the eye. Patients may have associated redness, although this should be mild and intermittent with dry eyes alone. Severe, deep pain associated with a dense red injection of the whites of the eye indicates possible scleritis—a condition warranting emergent referral to an ophthalmologist. Other possible causes of ocular pain are iritis/uveitis, angle closure glaucoma, recurrent erosions, eyelid mispositioning, or trigeminal neuralgia.

Varicella zoster is another important cause of ocular pain without antecedent trauma. Patients will complain of hemifacial pain that may precede vesicular formation characteristic of the disease. Lesions involving the nasal tip indicate nasociliary nerve involvement and increase the likelihood of ocular involvement.[8] Herpes zoster can affect every ocular structure, and signs of involvement or visual compromise should prompt urgent referral to an eye care provider.

### With trauma

Ocular trauma can be devastating to vision and must be carefully evaluated to avoid diagnostic error. Unfortunately, there is not a direct correlation between pain and severity of injury. A corneal abrasion can be severely painful but not sight threatening, whereas an occult globe rupture from metallic foreign body may be painless. In many cases, the mechanism of injury is the most important risk factor for severe injury. Metal on metal striking injuries along with projectiles and shattered glass have high incidences of globe laceration and highlight the importance of encouraging use of occupational safety glasses. High-risk recreational activities are personal fireworks, use of airsoft/BB guns, and paintball.

Examination findings that suggest severe ocular trauma include peaked pupils, gross blood in the eye, severe vision loss, and foreign body embedded in or near the eye. Any potential open-globe injuries should be treated with rigid shield protection, avoidance of ocular manipulation, and immediate referral for specialty evaluation. Although blunt injuries are less likely to cause ocular laceration, they commonly cause orbital floor fractures or hyphema. Hemodynamically stable patients with orbital floor fractures should be managed as an outpatient where persistent diplopia or cosmetic concerns may prompt fracture repair.

## Patients at Risk for Vision Loss

### Glaucoma

Glaucoma is most often a slowly progressive, painless ocular disease that leads to blindness. It is more common with increasing age. Primary care physicians can be critical to detecting these patients by screening their patients for risk factors. Patients should be encouraged to get their eyes checked, if they are not being followed-up by an optometrist or ophthalmologist, if they

- Are older than 40 years
- Have family members with glaucoma

- Are of African, Hispanic, or Asian heritage
- Have high eye pressure
- Had An eye injury
- Use long-term steroid medications
- Have diabetes
- Have migraines
- Have high blood pressure
- Have poor blood circulation
- Have other health problems affecting the whole body
- Have large optic nerve cupping

Patients with more than one of the risk factors are at even higher risk.

### Diabetic retinopathy

Primary care physicians are the greatest asset in reducing diabetic retinopathy and work with ophthalmologists to decrease blindness from this disease. Motivating patients to manage their disease is amazingly difficult, but disciplines working together are more effective. Finding referral physicians that work with the primary care doctor is essential to improve patient care. Patients with type 1 diabetes should have annual screenings beginning 5 years after onset of disease. Patients with type 2 diabetes should undergo screening at the time of diagnosis and annually thereafter.[9]

### Medication toxicity

Many different medications used to treat systemic conditions can have ocular side effects. This series of articles has an entire article that discusses systemic medications with potential ocular side effects, but several medications are highlighted here. Patients on the following medications have high rates of ocular toxicity and should be proactively evaluated by an ophthalmologist at initiation of treatment:

- *Ethambutol*: known to be toxic to optic nerve function. Can occur early in the course of treatment of mycobacterial disease and affects approximately 1% of all patients on the medication at World Health Organization–recommended dosing.[10]
- *Hydroxychloroquine*: known to be a dose-dependent potential toxin to the retina. Baseline screening followed by annual screening after 5 years of treatment can help prevent irreversible vision loss. Recommended daily doses should not exceed 5.0 mg/kg of real body weight. Even at recommended doses, risk of toxicity after 20 years of treatment is 20%.[11]
- *Pentosan polysulfate sodium*: recently identified cause of potentially irreversible retinal damage. Now carries a black box warning regarding retinal toxicity.[12]

### Examination Techniques for General Medical Care

#### Lid eversion

Everting the upper eyelid can be helpful to evaluate patients with foreign body sensation or corneal abrasion of unclear cause. Place topical anesthetic on the eye. Now lid eversion can be accomplished by asking the patient to look down, grasping the eye lashes and pulling the lid off the globe. Then place a cotton-tipped applicator stick against the upper edge of the tarsal plate to use as a fulcrum and pull the lid up as you gently press down with the applicator stick, everting the lid. Any patient with verti cally oriented corneal abrasions, which could be an indication of a foreign body under the lid, should have this maneuver performed (**Fig. 7**).

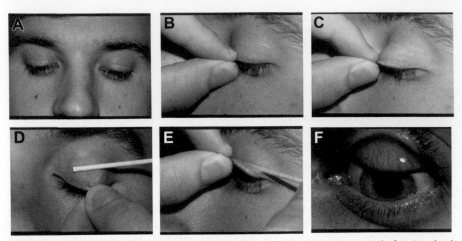

**Fig. 7.** Everting the upper eyelid can be helpful to evaluate patients with foreign body sensation or corneal abrasion of unclear etiology. Place topical anesthetic on the eye. (A & B) Now lid eversion can be accomplished by asking the patient to look down, grasping the eye lashes and pulling the lid off the globe. (C, D, E & F) Then place a cotton tipped applicator stick against the upper edge of the tarsal plate to use as a fulcrum and pull the lid up as you gently press down with the applicator stick, everting the lid. Any patient with vertically oriented corneal abrasions, which could be an indication of a foreign body under the lid, should have this maneuver performed.

### Fluorescein staining/cobalt blue light

Sodium fluorescein is an orange vital dye that stains areas of devitalized epithelium. When viewed under cobalt blue light such as with a Wood's lamp, areas of corneal abnormality will fluoresce, highlighting areas of corneal abrasion, dendritic ulceration, or foreign body. Focal, nonmobile areas of stain uptake should raise concern for ocular surface disease warranting referral for further evaluation (**Fig. 8**).

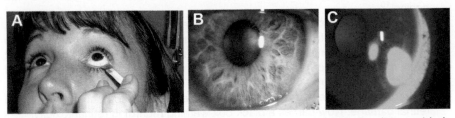

**Fig. 8.** Fluorescein staining is used to define corneal abrasion and other conditions with devitalized epithelium. First apply a topical ocular anesthetic to the eye. (A) Put an additional drop to the fluorescein strip, pull the inferior lid down, and apply the fluorescein drop at the edge of the lid and have the patient gently blink. (B) Stain alone will faintly outline the epithelial defect. (C) Next use a cobalt blue light to enhance the stain as seen in the photos.

### Check pupil response

Pupils should be assessed in a dimly lit room with the patient focusing on a distant target. The examiner should check for equality of size and reaction to light. Any anisocoria greater than 1 mm should be referred for evaluation. A bright, focused light source should be directed at each eye individually to illicit a brisk and symmetric

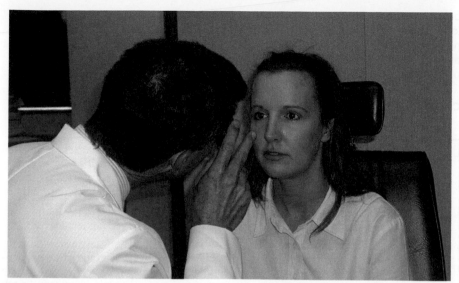

**Fig. 9.** The direct ophthalmoscope is useful for checking for red reflex and viewing the optic nerve and retina. The physician should use the right eye to examine the right eye and switch to the left eye to examine the left eye. Approach the patient about arm's length away and at about a 20° angle temporally, as the optic nerve will be at that location. Look at the red reflex then slowly move forward, focusing as you get closer to the eye. If the pupil is large enough and the red reflex clears, the optic nerve can be observed.

response. Swinging the focused light source from one eye to the other and back can be used to evaluate for a relative afferent pupillary defect wherein the effect eye will dilate rather than constrict.

### Direct ophthalmoscope
In a primary care office, direct ophthalmoscopy can be a time-consuming effort. Often times, dilation is required to view the optic nerve and retina adequately. Alternatively, using the direct ophthalmoscope to see if there is a clear red reflex in conjunction with patient history can help narrow down the diagnosis. For example, vision loss with pain

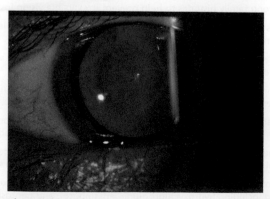

**Fig. 10.** In this dilated pupil the central red reflex is dim due to dense nuclear sclerosis of the lens. The view through this cataract would be very blurry and details of the optic nerve difficult to see.

on movement and a clear red reflex is more likely optic neuritis. Also, sudden vision loss with dull or no red reflex indicates there is media opacity, most likely vitreous hemorrhage or retinal detachment. If there is a clear red reflex, adequate pupil size, and you have the time, viewing the optic nerve is helpful in cases of vision loss, particularly those associated with headache or pain (**Figs. 9** and **10**).

## CLINICS CARE POINTS

- When a patient is suspected to have a recent stroke, confrontational visual fields should be performed at the initial evaluation if the patient is able to cooperate with the examination.
- When a patient has nonspecific visual complaints, visual acuity and confrontational visual fields should be performed.
- When a patient complains of irritated eyes, always ask exactly what drops (substances) they are putting in their eye and how often. Patients may be using products not suitable for the eyes or using eye drops excessively.
- On initial examination of a new patient ask if any family members are blind and why. Also ask if parents or siblings have been treated for glaucoma.
- Ask patients suspected to have multiple sclerosis if they have had any episodes of vision loss and ask them to describe the episodes.
- Patients will frequently assign allergies as the source of a red eye. To find the true cause, ask for them to describe symptoms, time course, and the over-the-counter treatments used.
- When seeing patients in the spring and summer, remind them to use goggles (not safety glasses) to protect their eyes when using a weed eater. Anyone else in the yard should also have goggles on.
- When seeing a patient for hand injury when using tools such as grinder or electric saw, ask if they use a protective eye goggles.
- Protective eyewear should be recommended for all patients engaging in high-risk activities such as metal grinding or construction, particularly for those who are monocular.
- The risk factors for glaucoma will be found in many patients older than 50 years. Remind patients to have their eyes checked, as several serious eye conditions are slowly progressive or even asymptomatic and if not detected early will result in permanent visual loss.
- Glaucoma is often asymptomatic until advance stages, and primary care providers should inquire about strong family histories to help prevent irreversible vision loss.
- Visual complaints are best evaluated in the context of the temporal profile of disease, with acute vision loss necessitating urgent referral.
- Double vision that is worse in certain directions of gaze and goes away with occlusion of either eye is more likely to be neurologic and requires further workup.
- Intense photophobia in conjunction with a red eye should raise concern for uveitis, particularly if there is a history of immune-mediated or infectious disease.
- Patients with viral conjunctivitis are highly contagious, and strict contact precautions should be taken by both the provider and the patient to avoid community spread.
- Dry eye syndrome is the most prevalent cause of ocular irritation and intermittent blurred vision, which typically responds to over-the-counter artificial tears as a first-line treatment.
- A wide variety of systemic medications have ocular side effects or toxicity that require vigilant screening including hydroxychloroquine, ethambutol, and pentosan.
- Ocular trauma can have devastating visual consequences and any patient presenting with decreased acuity after trauma should be thoroughly evaluated.

* Recurrent amaurosis, headache, scalp tenderness, and jaw claudication are among the many potential symptoms of GCA and require high index of clinical suspicion due to severe visual consequences of unrecognized disease.

## DISCLOSURE

The authors have nothing to disclose.

## REFERENCES

1. National Center for Health Statistics (US). Health, United States, 2010: With Special Feature on Death and Dying. Hyattsville (MD): National Center for Health Statistics (US); 2011 Feb. Report No.: 2011-1232. PMID: 21634072.
2. Shields T, Sloane PD. A comparison of eye problems in primary care and ophthalmology practices. Fam Med 1991;23(7):544–6.
3. Flaxel CJ, Adelman RA, Bailey ST, et al. Posterior vitreous detachment, retinal breaks, and lattice degeneration preferred practice pattern®. Ophthalmology 2020;127(1):P146–81.
4. Flaxel CJ, Adelman RA, Bailey ST, et al. Retinal and ophthalmic artery occlusions preferred practice pattern®. Ophthalmology 2020;127(2):P259–87.
5. Linda RD, Federico GV, Steven MA, et al. Adult strabismus preferred practice pattern®. Ophthalmology 2020;127(1):P182–298.
6. Azar MJ, Dhaliwal DK, Bower KS, et al. Possible consequences of shaking hands with your patients with epidemic keratoconjunctivitis. Am J Ophthalmol 1996; 121(6):711–2.
7. Doyle TJ, King D, Cobb J, et al. An outbreak of epidemic keratoconjunctivitis at an outpatient ophthalmology clinic. Infect Dis Rep 2010;2(2):e17.
8. Zaal MJW, Völker-Dieben HJ, D'Amaro J. Prognostic value of Hutchinson's sign in acute herpes zoster ophthalmicus. Graefes Arch Clin Exp Ophthalmol 2003; 241(3):187–91.
9. Flaxel CJ, Adelman RA, Bailey ST, et al. Diabetic retinopathy preferred practice pattern®. Ophthalmology 2020;127(1):P66–145.
10. Chamberlain PD, Sadaka A, Berry S, et al. Ethambutol optic neuropathy. Curr Opin Ophthalmol 2017;28(6):545–51.
11. Marmor MF, Kelner U, Lai TY, et al. Recommendations on screening for chloroquine and hydroxychloroquine retinopathy (2016 Revision). Ophthalmology 2016;123(6):1386–94.
12. Pentosan [package insert]. Titusville (NJ): Janssen Pharmaceuticals, Inc; 2020.

# Ocular Side Effects of Common Systemic Medications and Systemic Side Effects of Ocular Medications

Misha F. Syed, MD, MEHP*, Ahmad Rehmani, DO,
Matthew Yang, MD

## KEYWORDS

- Ocular topical medications • Ocular side effects • Medication • Eye • Eye drops
- Vision changes

## KEY POINTS

- Physicians should be aware of potential ocular side effects of systemic medications when prescribing therapy.
- Ocular medications may induce systemic side effects that could affect management of various conditions; therefore, knowing patients' ophthalmologic diagnoses and therapy can be useful.
- Treatment of ocular conditions may require topical and/or systemic medications, with implications for the overall health of patients.

## INTRODUCTION

We have organized this article into 2 main sections: ocular side effects of commonly prescribed drugs and systemic side effects of medications commonly prescribed by ophthalmologists. The article lists the class of drugs, their mechanism of action (MOA), known and possible ocular side effects (OSEs), and recommendations for OSEs to watch out for and/or medications that need ophthalmologic screening before or during use. For topical/ocular medications, the ocular and systemic side effects are discussed, as well as situations in which to avoid their use.

The reader is encouraged to consider these side effects when prescribing the following classes of medications and should be able to use this article as a reference when encountering a patient with visual symptoms, especially in the setting of possible ocular toxicity.

University of Texas Medical Branch, 700 University Boulevard, Galveston, TX 77555, USA
* Corresponding author.
E-mail address: mfsyed@utmb.edu

Med Clin N Am 105 (2021) 425–444
https://doi.org/10.1016/j.mcna.2021.02.003
0025-7125/21/© 2021 Elsevier Inc. All rights reserved.

**KEY POINTS**

- Hydroxychloroquine requires ongoing screening; toxicity risk increases with total lifetime (cumulative) dose, to some extent increased daily dose, and with concurrent tamoxifen use.
- Patients with current or past use of tamsulosin (and other alpha blockers) may develop floppy iris, which can complicate cataract surgery (intraoperative floppy iris syndrome).
- Corticosteroids often result in increased intraocular pressure and cataract formation, especially with prolonged use.
- Antihistamines can lead to dry eye syndrome.
- Statins may affect the ocular surface, lens, extraocular muscles, and retina.
- Isotretinoin may cause night blindness, pseudotumor cerebri.
- Various central nervous system drugs affect accommodation and near vision.
- Ethambutol can cause irreversible optic neuropathy.
- Tamoxifen deposition often presents on the cornea and the retina.
- Patients on topical beta blockers for glaucoma can have any systemic side effects of oral beta blockers.
- Anti-vascular endothelial growth factor injections are common in treatment of age-related macular degeneration, and present a small increased risk of thromboembolic events.
- Various chemotherapeutic agents can have a variety of ocular surface, retinal, and optic nerve toxicities.
- Medications instilled into the eye have the same potential side effects as when administered systemically, albeit often to a lesser degree.

## OCULAR SIDE EFFECTS OF COMMONLY PRESCRIBED MEDICATIONS
### Antimalarials

*Indications:* Antimalarial agents are also commonly prescribed to treat several rheumatic and skin conditions.

*Name/MOA:* Hydroxychloroquine (HCQ) and chloroquine (CQ). MOA not well-understood.

Known OSE:
- *Cornea*:
  - Diffuse punctate opacities, verticillate more with CQ than HCQ use.
  - Deposits rarely have visual sequelae and typically resolve on their own with or without discontinuation of treatment.
- *Retina*:
  - CQ and HCQ affect the outer layers of the retina, primarily the photoreceptors and retinal pigment epithelium.
  - "Bulls-eye" appearance on fundus examination; damage occurs in a ring around the fovea sparing its very center
  - At Risk: Dose and time dependent.
    - High risk: Cumulative daily dose of greater than 5 mg/kg of HCQ and greater than 2.3 mg/kg of CQ.
    - At recommended doses, risk of toxicity is less than 2% at 10 years, but rises sharply to 20% after 20 years.
    - Renal disease, tamoxifen use, and preexisting retinal or macular disease can also increase the risk of toxicity.

*Possible/Rare OSE:* Difficulty with accommodation and formation of cataracts.

Recommendations:
- Baseline ophthalmic examination within the first year if starting HCQ/CQ.
- Thereafter, annual ophthalmologic screenings can be deferred until 5 years of exposure if dosage is proper, or annually if high risk.
- 10 to 2 automated visual fields which focus on central vision and optical coherence tomography, which displays distinctive retinal layers should be done at all ophthalmology visits.

## Antiarrhythmics

*Indications:* To restore sinus rhythm in patients presenting with cardiac arrhythmias, as well as to prevent recurrent arrhythmias.
*Name/MOA:* Amiodarone: di-iodinated benzofuran derivative.

Known OSE:
- Vortex keratopathy (cornea verticillata); corneal microdeposits occurring in 70% to 100% of patients but usually does not cause decrease in vision.
- Anterior subcapsular lens opacities.
- Multiple chalazia (stylelike lesions on eyelids).
- Dry eye syndrome.
- Most serious ocular side effect is amiodarone-associated optic neuropathy, which can cause vision loss and may not resolve quickly or completely even with cessation of medication.

*Name/MOA:* Digoxin: Potent reversible inhibitor of cellular sodium potassium adenosine triphosphatase (Na/K ATPase), mainly in the myocardium.

Possible/rare OSE:
- Can cause optic neuropathy associated with vision loss, may not resolve quickly or completely even with cessation of medication. Potential dyschromatopsia (xanthopsia – yellow vision, cyanopsia – blue vision, chloropsia – green vision).

*Name/MOA:* Oxprenolol, propranolol: Beta adrenergic antagonists.

Known OSE:
- Decreased vision
- (Transient) diplopia
- Visual hallucinations
- Eyelid changes (erythema, urticaria, purpura)
- Lacrimation
- Photophobia
- Decreased intraocular pressure (IOP)
Possible/rare OSE:
- Myasthenia gravis, decreased accommodation, inflammatory intraocular pseudotumor, exfoliative dermatitis of lids

*Name/MOA:* Quinidine: Blocks sodium and potassium currents across cellular membranes, prolongs cellular action potential and decreases automaticity.

Known OSE:
- Visual disturbance
Possible/rare OSE:
- Color vision defect (red-green), photosensitivity, eyelid changes (urticaria, edema, lupoid syndrome), anterior granulomatous uveitis, visual hallucinations, ocular sicca (may aggravate or cause condition), myasthenia gravis, corneal deposits

## Anticoagulants

*Indications:* prophylaxis and/or treatment of thromboembolic events such as cerebrovascular accident, pulmonary embolism, and myocardial infarction.
*Name/MOA:* warfarin: vitamin K epoxide reductase inhibitor.
*Name/MOA:* heparin: activation of antithrombin III and inactivation of thrombin.
*Name/MOA:* apixaban: direct inhibitor of factor Xa.

Known OSE:
- Hemorrhages
  - Within any ocular or peribulbar structures (retinal, orbital, choroidal, vitreous, retrobulbar, subretinal, hyphema).
  - Often associated with complications after recent ocular surgery.
  - One study estimated the prevalence of warfarin-associated ocular hemorrhage at approximately 3%.[1–7]
  - Novel oral anticoagulants possibly safer or equal in risk of intraocular hemorrhage.
  - Treatment: likely sufficient to temporary pause therapy, however surgical intervention may be needed.[8,9]

Recommendations:
- Complications vary from case to case and have a wide range in severity and effects on vision and ocular structures.
- Each case must be individualized depending on the location of hemorrhage and structures threatened.
- Stopping anticoagulant therapy can often lead to more devastating outcomes from systemic disease.

## Antidepressants

*Indications:* To treat various types of clinical depression and/or anxiety disorders. May be prescribed off-label to treat other conditions not approved by the Food and Drug Administration (FDA).
*Name/MOA:* Amitriptyline, clomipramine, doxepin, trimipramine: Tricyclic antidepressants (tertiary amine)/serotonin-norepinephrine reuptake inhibitors.

Known OSE:
- Mydriasis
- Potential for acute glaucoma in predisposed persons
- Decreased accommodation/blurred vision
- Ocular sicca (may aggravate or cause condition)
- Decreased contact lens tolerance

Possible/rare OSE:
- Blepharospasm, oculogyric crisis, nystagmus (with toxicity)

*Name/MOA:* Atomoxetine, duloxetine, venlafaxine: serotonin-norepinephrine reuptake inhibitors

Known OSE:
- Mydriasis
- Decreased vision
- Potential for acute glaucoma in predisposed persons

Possible/rare OSE:
- Ocular sicca (may aggravate or cause condition), cataracts, visual hallucinations, photophobia, eyelid edema, blepharospasm

*Name/MOA:* Bupropion HCl: Aminoketone.

Known OSE:
- Weak mydriasis
- Decreased vision
- Visual hallucinations

Possible/rare OSE:
- Myopia, ocular sicca (may aggravate or cause condition), diplopia, eyelid edema, periorbital edema, may precipitate acute glaucoma.

Name/MOA:
   Citalopram, escitalopram, fluoxetine, fluvoxamine, paroxetine, sertraline: selective serotonin reuptake inhibitors

Known OSE:
- Decreased vision
- Photophobia
- Ocular sicca (may aggravate or cause condition)
- Non–rapid eye movement during sleep

Possible/rare OSE:
- Oculogyric crisis, pupil changes (mydriasis, anisocoria), optic neuritis, ischemic optic neuropathy, cataracts/lens opacities

*Name/MOA:* Isocarboxazid, phenelzine, tranylcypromine: monoamine oxidase inhibitors (MAOIs)

Known OSE:
- Decreased vision
- Visual hallucinations (phenelzine)

Possible/rare OSE:
- Diplopia, nystagmus, strabismus, myasthenia gravis, photophobia, color vision defect (red-green)

*Name/MOA:* Trazodone: Triazolopyridine derivative, MOA not fully understood: serotonin reuptake inhibitor, histamine and alpha-1-adrenergic receptor blocker, affects 5-HT presynaptic receptor adrenoreceptors.

Known OSE:
- Decreased vision
- Weak mydriasis
- Potential for acute glaucoma in predisposed persons
- Visual distortions including metallic ghost images, bright shiny lights, palinopsia

Possible/rare OSE:
- Ocular sicca (may aggravate or cause condition), photosensitivity, blepharoconjunctivitis, diplopia

### Antihypertensives

*Indications:* Reduction of blood pressure in hypertension, control of tachyarrhythmias, prevention of cardiac remodeling, and diuresis in congestive heart failure.

*Name/MOA:* Beta blockers: selective or nonselective inhibitors of the beta (and alpha) adrenergic receptors.

Known OSE:
- Systemic beta blockers
  - Low IOP
  - Transitory decreased vision
  - Hallucinations

o Dry eye symptoms

*Name/MOA:* Angiotensin-converting enzyme (ACE) inhibitors: compete for ACE to reduce levels of angiotensin II.

Known OSE:
- ACE inhibitors
  o Conjunctivitis
  o Periorbital edema
  o Facial urticaria

*Name/MOA:* Thiazides: inhibit sodium reabsorption of the renal distal tubules.

Known OSE:
- Thiazides
  o Decreased vision
  o Color defects
  o Acute angle closure glaucoma (AACG)
  o Band keratopathy secondary to hypercalcemia
Possible/rare OSE:
- Retinal phototoxicity, macular edema

## Alpha Blockers

*Indications:* Benign prostatic hyperplasia, hypertension, Raynaud disease, and erectile dysfunction.
*Name/MOA:* Tamsulosin, Alfuzosin, Doxazosin, Prazosin, Terazosin, Silodosin: Blockage of alpha receptors leads to smooth muscle relaxation.

### Known OSE
### IFIS (intraoperative floppy iris syndrome)
- The iris dilator muscle, a smooth muscle with predominance of alpha-1A receptors, functions to regulate pupillary size. As the iris is anterior to the human lens, pupillary dilation is imperative for visualization to perform cataract extraction and intraocular lens insertion.
- Systemic alpha-1 receptor blockade can result in significant loss of iris tone resulting in IFIS.
- Triad of:
  o Pupillary constriction intraoperatively despite preoperative pharmacologic dilation
  o Fluttering and bellowing of iris stroma
  o Tendency of iris to prolapse toward side port incisions during surgery
- Occurrence: Within days of starting medication or even 1-time use can result in IFIS; stopping the medication before cataract surgery does not prevent IFIS, and even remote history of medication use can cause IFIS years later.
Recommendations:
- Operative strategies as well as pharmacologic and mechanical devices have helped to reduce the complications of IFIS.
- Physicians should refer patient for evaluation of cataracts (if they have not already had cataract surgery) before starting medications in this class (all alpha receptor blocking medications) whenever possible. This will allow the patient to have cataract surgery if indicated before being on the medication and therefore lessen risk of IFIS.

## Antihistamines

*Indication:* Allergic relief, anaphylactic reactions, and drug-induced extrapyramidal symptoms.

*Name/MOA:* Diphenhydramine, cetirizine, loratadine: direct competitor to histamine at H1-receptor sites.

Known OSE:

- Mydriasis
- Decreased vision
- Decreased light reflex
- Decreased contact lens tolerance
- Anisocoria
- AACG[10–16]

## Diuretics

*Indications:* To treat hypertension, chronic edema secondary to congestive heart failure, and cirrhosis. May also be used to help prevent calcium kidney stones to treat nephrogenic diabetes insipidus.

*Name/MOA:* Carbonic anhydrase inhibitors (CAI): Inhibition of carbonic anhydrase, which is present in the ciliary body epithelium reduces the formation of bicarbonate ions, which reduces fluid transport, thus reducing IOP. Other proposed mechanisms include vascular dilation to the optic nerve. CAIs also specifically used for altitude sickness prophylaxis and treatment of idiopathic intracranial hypertension. CAIs may have other off-label, non–FDA-approved uses.

Oral CAIs are often used either alone or in conjunction with topical glaucoma therapy to treat elevated IOP chronically. They may also be used to acutely lower IOP, commonly before/after intraocular surgery or in cases of AACG.

Known OSE:

- Inhibition of carbonic anhydrase, which is present in the ciliary body epithelium reduces the formation of bicarbonate ions, which reduces fluid transport, thus reducing IOP.
- Rarely, use of CAIs (sulfonamide derivative) can result in ciliochoroidal effusion syndrome, which causes an acute bilateral angle closure. Cessation of the CAI is the main treatment for this condition, which generally resolves after discontinuation.

Recommendations:

- As diuretics rid the body of excess fluids, they also may lead to decreased tear production regardless of class or type. Artificial tears may be beneficial in symptomatic patients.
- In sickle cell disease, metabolic acidosis due to CAI use can induce sickling. Special caution is advised if using CAIs to treat elevated IOP in patients with sickle cell disease (even patients with sickle cell trait), particularly those with a hyphema, as this can lead to anterior segment ischemia and even central retinal artery occlusion.

*Name/MOA:* Mineralocorticoid antagonists (MA) are potassium-sparing diuretics used to treat hypertension.

Known OSE:

- Use as diuretics has prompted investigation into therapy for several retinal diseases. Specifically, patients with central serous retinopathy have shown resolution of subretinal fluid. There have been rare reports of eplerenone use leading to uveal effusion syndrome.

### Erectile Dysfunction Drugs

*Indication:* Medications used to treat erectile dysfunction and (at higher doses) pulmonary hypertension.

*Name/MOA:* Sildenafil, tadalafil: phosphodiesterase-5 inhibition leading to buildup of cyclic guanosine monophosphate.

Known OSE:
- Color defects
- Light sensitivity
- Minimal hazy vision

Possible/rare OSE:
- Nonarteritic anterior ischemic optic neuropathy (NAION)
  - Although rare, this event may cause irreversible vision loss
  - Risk factors identified include men older than 50, hypertension, diabetes, and dyslipidemia

Recommendations:
- Return precautions for hazy vision or vision loss, especially for patients with risk factors for NAION
- Cessation of offending agent and immediate ophthalmologic evaluation in the event of sudden vision loss

### Nonsteroidal Anti-inflammatory Drugs

*Indications:* To relieve pain and fever, reduce inflammation.

*MOA:* Cyclooxygenase-1 (COX-1) and cyclooxygenase-2 (COX-2) inhibitors.

Known OSE:
- Corneal opacities
- Macular/retinal pigmentary changes (indomethacin: long-term use, no clear relationship to dosage and retinal toxicity)
- Vortex keratopathy
- Photosensitivity
- Orbital/periorbital/eyelid edema

Possible/rare OSE:
- Ocular sicca (may aggravate or cause condition), optic or retrobulbar neuritis, papilledema secondary to pseudotumor cerebri

### Proton Pump Inhibitors

Not known to cause significant OSEs.

### Corticosteroids

*Indication:* To treat inflammatory conditions, autoimmune diseases, allergic reactions, adrenocortical insufficiency.

*Name/MOA:* Betamethasone, budesonide, dexamethasone, fludrocortisone, fluorometholone, beclomethasone, fluticasone, hydrocortisone, prednisone, prednisolone, triamcinolone: Effects are systemic and widespread including decreasing inflammation and immune system activity, suppressing polymorphonuclear lymphocytes migration, stabilizing leukocyte release of hydrolases, and reversing capillary permeability.

*Known OSE*
**Systemic applications (via oral, intravenous, intramuscular, intra-articular, intranasal routes)**
- Decreased vision
- Increased IOP
- Pseudotumor cerebri
- Cataract formation
- Decreased resistance to infections
- Mydriasis leading to AACG (in predisposed persons)
- Visual field defects
- Retinal edema
- Retinal hemorrhage
- Central serous retinopathy

**Inhalant or topical applications**
- Increased IOP
- Decreased resistance to infections
- Pseudotumor cerebri
- Cataract formation

## Statins

*Indications:* Lipid-lowering drugs with anti-inflammatory, vascular, and immunomodulatory properties used primarily as cholesterol-lowering therapy.

*Name/MOA:* Pravastatin, atorvastatin, fluvastatin, lovastatin, pitavastatin, rosuvastatin, simvastatin. 3-hydroxy-3-methylglutaryl-coenzyme (HMG-CoA) reductase inhibitors.

Possible OSE:
- *Lens*: Interference with normal cholesterol accumulation in lens fibers and production of oxide derivatives leading to eventual cataract formation
- *Glaucoma*: Inhibition of rho-kinase and upregulation of nitric oxide leading to increased aqueous humor outflow, which lowers IOP
- *Dry eyes/Ocular inflammatory disease*: Blockage of inflammatory markers that break down the ocular surface
- *Orbital Myositis*: Extraocular muscles may be targets of the well-known statin side effects of muscle breakdown
- *Age-related Macular Degeneration (AMD)*: Reduction of inflammation, stabilization of the retinal pigment epithelium, which is the main target of macular degeneration
- *Diabetes*: Reduction of inflammatory markers and vascular endothelial growth factor (VEGF) leading to prevention of progression in diabetic retinopathy

## Antidiabetic Drugs

*Indication:* Antidiabetic medications used to lower serum glucose levels.
*Name/MOA:* Sulfonylureas: stimulate pancreatic release of insulin.

Known OSE:
- Tolbutamide: color deficiencies, most commonly blue-yellow impairment
- Glyburide: decreased accommodation, color deficiencies
- Osmotic lens changes
Possible/rare OSE:
- Optic neuritis or retrobulbar neuritis

*Name/MOA:* Metformin: decreases hepatic glucose production, decreases intestinal absorption of glucose, and improves insulin sensitivity by increasing peripheral glucose uptake and utilization.

- Not known to cause significant OSEs.

Recommendations:

- Drug-induced OSEs may be difficult to distinguish, as diabetes has many ocular manifestations.
- Diabetic patients should be monitored regularly with diabetic fundus examinations.

## OCULAR SIDE EFFECTS OF LESS COMMONLY PRESCRIBED SYSTEMIC MEDICATIONS
### Anemia Medications

Not known to cause significant OSEs.

### Anti-anginal Medications

*Indications:* For the relief of angina caused by cerebral and peripheral ischemia, associated with arterial spasm and myocardial ischemia (possibly complicated by cardiac arrhythmias).
*Name/MOA:* Nitroglycerin: relaxation of vascular smooth muscle.

Possible/Rare OSE:

- Has rarely been linked to decreased vision, colored halos, variations in IOP, and pseudotumor cerebri.

### Antiemetics

First-line antiemetics such as ondansetron are not known to affect ocular function. Antipsychotics with antiemetic action such as chlorpromazine and parasympathetic drugs are covered in another section.

### Antiretroviral Medications

*Indications:* To manage and treat human immunodeficiency virus (HIV)/AIDS infection, to prevent HIV infection transfer.

Name/MOA:
    Abacavir, didanosine, emtricitabine, lamivudine, stavudine, tenofovir, zidovudine: nucleoside reverse transcriptase inhibitors (NRTIs).
    Delavirdine, doravirine, efavirenz, etravirine, nevirapine, rilpivirine: non-NRTIs
    Atazanavir, darunavir, fosamprenavir, indinavir, lopinavir, nelfinavir, ritonavir, saquinavir, tipranavir: protease inhibitors
    Enfuvirtide: fusion inhibitors
    Maraviroc: CC chemokine receptor 5 antagonists
    Bictegravir, dolutegravir, elvitegravir, raltegravir: integrase inhibitors
    Fostemsavir: attachment inhibitors
    Ibalizumab: postattachment inhibitors
    Cobicistat: pharmacokinetic enhancers
    Possible OSE (reported with didanosine):

- Peripheral chorioretinal degeneration, which may be progressive despite cessation of medication, immune recovery uveitis including cystoid macular edema/epiretinal membranes/optic disc neovascularization

## Bisphosphonates

*Indications:* To treat and/or prevent osteoporosis from various causes, including post-menopausal state in women, osteoporosis in men, glucocorticoid-induced osteoporosis, Paget disease of bone.

*Name/MOA:* Alendronate/cholecalciferol, etidronate, zoledronic acid, risedronate, ibandronate, pamidronate, tiludronate. Inhibitors of osteoclast-mediated bone resorption.

Possible/rare OSE:
- Conjunctivitis, episcleritis, scleritis, uveitis

## H2 Blockers

*Indications:* To treat dyspepsia, peptic ulcers, gastroesophageal reflux disease, prevention of stress ulcers (specifically ranitidine), prevention of aspiration pneumonitis during surgery (oral formulation).

*Names/MOA:* Ranitidine, famotidine, cimetidine, nizatidine. Reversible binding to histamine H2 receptors on gastric parietal cells; function as competitive antagonists.

Possible/rare OSE:
- Retinal vascular occlusion, optic neuropathy, retrobulbar optic neuritis.

## Isotretinoin

*Indications:* Dermatologic conditions such as severe nodular acne and psoriasis.

*Name/MOA:* Isotretinoin is a synthetic vitamin A derivative that regulates epithelial proliferation and differentiation thereby inhibiting sebaceous gland function.

Known OSE:
- Night blindness (nyctalopia)
  - Slows regeneration of rhodopsin leading to retinal dysfunction
- Pseudotumor cerebri
  - May be due to alteration of lipid composition in arachnoid villi
- Blepharoconjunctivitis
  - Direct decrease of Meibomian gland function and secretion of drug via tears

Possible/rare OSE:
- Optic neuritis

Recommendations:
- Baseline dilated fundus examination could be useful before starting therapy
- Annual ophthalmologic examinations while on therapy, referral for any visual complaints while on therapy

## Opioid Analgesics (Narcotics)

*Indications:* To provide pain relief, including anesthesia. Can also be used to reverse opioid overdose, as replacement therapy for opioid use disorder, and to suppress cough.

*Name/MOA:* Fentanyl: Phenylpiperidine synthetic opiate agonist.

Known OSE:
- Miosis
- Visual hallucinations
- Oculogyric crisis

Possible/rare OSE:
- Extraocular muscle abnormalities (ptosis, diplopia, abnormal eye movements), eyelid edema, periorbital edema

*Name/MOA:* Hydromorphone, oxymorphone: hydrogenated ketones of morphine.

Known OSE:
- Decreased vision
- Decreased accommodation
- Miosis
- Eyelid changes (urticaria, contact dermatitis)

Possible/rare OSE:
- Extraocular muscle abnormalities (nystagmus, diplopia), visual hallucinations.

*Name/MOA:* Meperidine: phenylpiperidine narcotic analgesic.

Known OSE:
- Miosis
- Decreased vision
- Eyelid changes (erythema, urticaria)
- Visual hallucinations

Possible/rare OSE:
- Nystagmus, ocular signs of drug-induced Parkinson disease (ptosis, diplopia, paresis/paralysis of extraocular muscles)

*Name/MOA:* Methadone: synthetic analgesic.

Known OSE:
- Miosis
- Talc retinopathy (with intravenous use)
- Decreased vision
- Decreased spontaneous eye movements

Possible/rare OSE:
- Eyelid changes (urticaria, edema), ocular sicca (may aggravate or cause condition), extraocular muscle abnormalities (diplopia, nystagmus, strabismus), cerebral visual impairment, reduced visual evoked potential

*Name/MOA:* Morphine sulfate:

Known OSE:
- Miosis
- Decreased vision
- Extraocular muscle abnormalities (diplopia, nystagmus, decreased convergence)
- Decreased accommodation
- Decreased IOP
- Visual hallucinations
- Decreased lacrimation
- Eyelid changes (urticaria, pruritis)
- Color vision defect (mainly blue-yellow, usually with chronic abuse)
- Ptosis

Possible/rare OSE:
- Myopia, ocular sicca (may aggravate or cause condition), accommodative spasm, vertical nystagmus, potential teratogenic effect of strabismus in exposed fetuses

*Name/MOA:* Pentazocine, Naloxone: benzomorphan narcotic analgesic.

Known OSE:
- Miosis

- Decreased vision
- Visual hallucinations

Possible/rare OSE:

- Nystagmus, diplopia, decreased accommodation, eyelid changes (erythema, edema), decreased spontaneous eye movements, oculogyric crisis

## Tuberculosis Drugs

*Name:* Ethambutol, isoniazid, rifampicin, and streptomycin: common drugs used for treatment of mycobacterium tuberculosis (TB).

MOA:
  Ethambutol: mechanism not completely understood
  Isoniazid: prodrug that inhibits formation of mycobacterial cell wall
  Rifampicin: inhibits bacterial RNA polymerase
  Streptomycin: protein synthesis inhibitor
Known OSE:
  Ethambutol-induced optic neuropathy
- Optic neuropathy be related to deficiency of copper, zinc, or vitamins E and B1.
- Symptoms: bilateral in more than 60% of patients.
  - Visual acuity loss ranging from 20/25 to no light perception
  - Visual field defects commonly involving central or cecocentral scotomas
  - Dyschromatopsia primarily affecting red/green vision and to a lesser degree blue/yellow loss
- Incidence: dose dependent: less than 1% with 15 mg/kg increasing to 18% to 33% with greater than 35 mg/kg per day
- At risk: hypertension, age older than 65, renal disease
- *Treatment*: Discontinuation of ethambutol. However, damage is often irreversible, as only 30% to 64% of patients report visual improvement.
Isoniazid:
- Can rarely cause retrobulbar optic neuritis especially in combination with ethambutol
Rifampicin:
- Staining of bodily fluids, particularly sweat and tears, to an orange-red color is common and may even be used to monitor absorption of the drug.
- Tears may permanently stain soft contact lenses but does not require medical attention.
Streptomycin:
- Can cause pseudotumor cerebri and myasthenic neuromuscular blockade. Should be avoided in patients with myasthenia gravis and anesthesia with neuromuscular blocking agents.

*Recommendations:* Baseline ophthalmic examination before initiation of anti-TB drugs and continued ophthalmic examinations during treatment as indicated.

## Antiepileptics

*Indication:* Treatment of epilepsy and various headache disorders.
*Name/MOA:* Topiramate: Sulfonamide drug known to affect multiple targets including inhibition of voltage-gated sodium channels, enhancement of GABA-A receptors, and mild inhibition of carbonic anhydrase isoenzymes.

Known/uncommon OSE:
  Ciliochoroidal effusion syndrome

- Sulfa derivatives known to cause lenticular swelling and forward displacement of iris-lens diaphragm resulting in forward rotation of ciliary body
- Presentation may mimic that of migraine headaches (headache, nausea, vomiting), but will typically include vision loss, hyperemia, corneal edema
- AACG most common and concerning adverse effect that typically occurs 7.0 to 12.8 days from administration (but can occur weeks after administration of drug)
- Acute myopia may develop within hours or weeks of starting therapy
- Treatment: cessation of offending agent, topical and systemic IOP-lowering medications to manage IOP acutely

Recommendations:

- Immediate cessation of topiramate and alternative therapy for the preexisting systemic pathology
- Prompt ophthalmologic evaluation for AACG to mitigate irreversible loss
- Acute myopia is often resolved within days but may take weeks for resolution in some cases

### Pentosan Polysulfate Sodium (Elmiron)

*Indications:* To treat bladder pain/discomfort associated with interstitial cystitis.

*MOA:* Unknown; heparinlike macromolecular carbohydrate derivative resembling glycosaminoglycans.

Known OSE:

- Associated with retinal pigmentary changes (pigmentary maculopathy), cumulative dose-related so more common after more than 3 years of use. Changes may be irreversible; changes may also progress even after cessation of treatment.

Recommendations:

- Baseline retinal examination recommended within 6 months of starting therapy and periodically while continuing therapy.

## OCULAR SIDE EFFECTS OF ONCOLOGIC/IMMUNOMODULATORY MEDICATIONS
### Fingolimod

*Indications:* Oral therapy for relapsing, remitting multiple sclerosis (MS)

*Name/MOA:* Fingolimod: acts as an immune modulator that prevents binding of Sphingosine 1-phosphate to its receptor in lymphocytes; the primary cellular targets in MS.

Known OSE:

Fingolimod-associated macular edema (FAME)

- Interaction between fingolimod and retinal vascular endothelial cells is thought to decrease cellular adhesion and therefore increase vascular permeability resulting in macular edema.
- Symptoms: asymptomatic to decreased visual acuity and metamorphopsias
- Incidence: 0.4% in patients treated with 0.5 mg and 1% in those treated with 1.25 mg of fingolimod. All reported cases of FAME occurred within the first 4 to 6 months of starting treatment.
- At risk: History of uveitis, diabetic retinopathy, or other ocular comorbidities
- Treatment: Discontinuation of fingolimod leads to cessation of FAME in 85% of patients. Remaining patients may benefit from steroid therapy.

Possible/Rare OSE:

- Retinal hemorrhages and retinal vein occlusions

Recommendations:

- If patients have no ocular comorbidities, an initial vision should be documented by providers and baseline dilated ophthalmic examination should be done within 3 to 4 months.
- If history of previously mentioned risk factors, ophthalmic examination should precede initiation of medication to discern if patient is a good candidate for therapy.

### Tamoxifen

*Indications:* An adjuvant treatment of patients with hormone-receptor positive breast cancer.

*MOA:* Tamoxifen is a selective estrogen receptor modulator.

Known OSE:
- *Cornea*: Cornea verticillate, a whorl like pattern, occurs due to the drug's resistance to enzymatic degradation once bound to lipids within the cornea. These lesions are rarely visually significant and usually do not require treatment.
- *Retina*: Crystalline deposits, macular edema and punctate pigmentary changes.
  - Symptoms: Decreased visual acuity and color vision.
  - At risk: Obesity, dyslipidemia, and dosage of medication. High doses (60–100 mg/d) may manifest as early as 1 year after initiation, whereas lower doses (10–20 mg/d) may take several years to present.
  - Incidence: 12% of patients
  - Treatment: Visual function and macular edema improve after drug cessation; however, crystal deposits do not immediately disappear. Persistent macular edema may be treated by anti-VEGF, corticosteroids, or CAIs.

*Recommendations:* All patients started on tamoxifen should be referred to an ophthalmologist for baseline evaluation and regular examinations while on treatment.

## TOPICAL/OPHTHALMIC MEDICATIONS WITH IMPORTANT SYSTEMIC SIDE EFFECTS

Ophthalmologists prescribe medications to treat a wide variety of ocular disorders.

The volume of commercial drop dispensers (approximately 25–50 μL) is generally greater than the capacity of the conjunctival sac. When drops are instilled, only 10% of the medication is absorbed. Smaller lipophilic drugs go through the cornea, whereas larger hydrophilic drugs traverse the conjunctiva/sclera. Fifty percent or more of this absorbed dose makes its way to the systemic circulation. Although medications given topically do not reach as high a concentration in the blood, any of the eye drops can have systemic absorption with systemic side effects. Thus, what may seem as a relatively benign amount of medication may cause significant systemic toxicity. The following are common topical medications and their potential systemic side effects.

### Topical Anesthetics

*Indications:* Used in everyday practice to numb the ocular surface before dilating drops, intravitreal injections, removal of surface corneal bodies, and much more.

*Name/MOA:* Tetracaine, proparacaine, lidocaine, oxybuprocaine: decrease neuronal membrane permeability to sodium ions, thus blocking initiation and conduction of nerve impulses.

- *Local side effects*: Temporary anesthesia. However, anesthetic abuse can lead to significant irreversible corneal damage and breakdown.
- *Recommendation*: Should not be prescribed to patients as an at-home medication.

## Mydriatics

*Indications:* Induce pupillary dilation. Several diagnostic and therapeutic indications, such as obtaining refraction, dilated fundus examinations, uveitis, amblyopia penalization, and treatment of accommodative esotropia.

*Name/MOA:* Atropine, scopolamine, homatropine, cyclopentolate, tropicamide: paralyze the ciliary body.

- *Local side effects*: Burning, photophobia, ocular irritation, eyelid edema, hyperemia, increased IOP, conjunctivitis
- *Systemic side effects:* Dry mouth/skin, behavioral disturbances, tachycardia, disorientation, seizures, hypotension, psychosis, respiratory depression, fever
- *Avoid in:* Elderly individuals, intraocular inflammation

*Name/MOA:* Phenylephrine: adrenergic receptor agonist

- *Local side effects*: Burning/stinging, pigmented aqueous floaters
- *Systemic side effects:* Rare: systemic hypertension, ventricular arrhythmia, tachycardia, subarachnoid hemorrhage
- *Avoid in:* Patients taking MAOIs, tricyclic antidepressants (TCAs), antidepressants, reserpine, guanethidine, methyldopa

## Intraocular Pressure–Lowering Agents

*Indications*: Glaucoma, lowering of IOP after intraocular surgery.

*Name/MOA:* Apraclonidine, Brimonidine: alpha agonists.

Alpha-1 activity: vasoconstriction, pupillary dilation, eyelid retraction.

Alpha-2 activity: Reduce aqueous production, increase aqueous outflow.

- *Local side effects*: Follicular conjunctivitis, contact dermatitis
- *Systemic side effects:* Dry mouth, allergy
- *Avoid in:* Pediatric patients due to central nervous system effects: risk of somnolence, hypotension, seizures, apnea. Patients taking MAOIs or TCAs.

*Name/MOA:* Timolol, betaxolol, levobunolol, metipranolol: beta blockers reduce aqueous production.

- *Local side effects*: Urticaria, alopecia, contact dermatitis, psoriasiform rashes
- *Systemic side effects:* Bradycardia, arrhythmias, syncope, hypotension, bronchoconstriction
- *Avoid in:* Patients with lung disease, patients already on oral therapy

*Name/MOA:* Dorzolamide, Brinzolamide: CAIs reduce aqueous production.

- *Local side effects*: Bitter aftertaste, eye burning/stinging, allergic conjunctival reaction, superficial punctate keratopathy
- *Systemic side effects:* Nausea. Of note, topical CAIs produce fewer side effects than oral treatment. Should be used with caution in patients with sickle cell disease.
- *Avoid in:* Sulfonamide allergy

*Name/MOA:* Pilocarpine, Carbachol: parasympathetics increase aqueous outflow by contraction of ciliary body, no longer first line for glaucoma.

- *Local side effects*: Pupillary constriction allergic dermatitis
- *Systemic side effects:* Excessive sweating, bronchospasm, vomiting, diarrhea, bradycardia, hypotension, confusion, emotional liability, agitation, concentration/behavioral disorders

- *Avoid in:* Patients with concurrent ocular inflammation.

*Name/MOA:* Common: Latanoprost, bimatoprost, tafluprost, travoprost, latanoprostene. Prostaglandin analogs increase aqueous outflow.

- *Local side effects*: Increased pigmentation of iris (irreversible), periorbital tissues (eyelids), and eyelashes (reversible). Elongates and thickens eyelashes. Burning, stinging, itching, increased lacrimation from irritation.
- *Systemic side effects:* Minimal. Use with caution during pregnancy (Class C: could stimulate uterine contractions leading to premature labor).
- *Avoid in:* Patients with concurrent ocular inflammation.

### Nonsteroidal Anti-inflammatory Drugs/Steroids

*Indications:* Anti-inflammatory, anti-analgesic. Used postoperatively and for cystoid macular edema, episcleritis, and other mild ocular inflammatory disorders. Steroids can be instilled as drops, ointment, injected around the eye, or intravitreally as an implant.

*Name/MOA:* Common: Acular, Acuvail, bromday, bromsite, ilevro, Nevanac, ocufen, proflensa, voltaren, Xibrom. Nonsteroidal anti-inflammatory and anti-analgesic properties.

- *Local side effects*: Rare allergic contact dermatitis
- *Systemic side effects:* Rarely: Asthma, gastrointestinal effects[4,12,17–54]

*Name/MOA:* Fluorometholone, loteprednol, rimexolone, prednisolone, difluprednate: Steroid medications of varying potency.

- *Local side effects*: Cataract, elevated IOP. Rarely allergic reactions.
- *Systemic side effects:* Minimal.

### Antibiotics

*Indications:* Bacterial conjunctivitis, postoperative, postinjury infection prophylaxis, corneal ulcers, intraocular infections.

*Name/MOA:* Moxifloxacin, ciprofloxacin, levofloxacin, ofloxacin, besifloxacin, gatifloxacin, azithromycin, gentamicin, tobramycin, erythromycin, bacitracin, polymyxin B-trimethoprim, neomycin-polymyxin B-gramicidin, neomycin-polymyxin B-bacitracin, bacitracin-polymyxin B, sulfacetamide: Various MOAs: either bactericidal or bacteriostatic.

- *Local side effects*: Burning/itching, skin irritation, anaphylaxis, delayed corneal wound healing. Intravitreal vancomycin can be toxic to the retina.
- *Systemic side effects:* Minimal.
- *Avoid in:* Patients with systemic allergies to the same class(es) of antibiotics.

### Ophthalmic Injections

Besides topical administration, some ocular medications are administered via injection into the subconjunctival space or vitreous cavity.

*Indications*: Antibiotics for infection, anti- VEGF agents for treatment of various conditions (listed in the next section), steroids for intraocular inflammation.

- *Local side effects*: Conjunctival hemorrhage, eye pain, cataract, vitreous floaters, IOP elevation, vitreous detachment, retinal detachment, endophthalmitis.
- *Avoid in:* Acute blepharitis/ocular surface infection, scleritis.

### Anti-Vascular Endothelial Growth Factor Agents

*Indications:* To help halt growth of abnormal neovascular proliferation in the treatment of wet AMD, diabetic retinopathy, retinal vein occlusion, neovascular glaucoma, macular edema. Some of these uses are off-label for certain medications.

*Name/MOA:* Common: Bevacizumab, aflibercept, Lucentis, brolucizumab. Anti-VEGF agents.

- *Local side effects:* See preceding section, "Ophthalmic Injections."
- *Systemic side effects:* Arterial thromboembolic event, myocardial infarction, stroke, venous thrombotic event, transient ischemic attack, hypertension.
- *Avoid in:* Patients at increased risk of thromboembolic events.

## DISCLOSURE

None of the authors has any financial or commercial conflicts of interest to disclose.

## REFERENCES

1. Costedoat-Chalumeau N, Dunogué B, Leroux G, et al. A critical review of the effects of hydroxychloroquine and chloroquine on the eye. Clin Rev Allergy Immunol 2015;49(3):317–26.
2. Yam JCS, Kwok AKH. Ocular toxicity of hydroxychloroquine. Hong Kong Med J 2006;12(4):294–304.
3. Marmor MF, Kellner U, Lai TY, et al. Recommendations on screening for chloroquine and hydroxychloroquine retinopathy. Ophthalmology 2016;123(6):1386–94.
4. Fraunfelder FT, Fraunfelder RW, editors. Drug-induced ocular side effects. 8th edition. New York: Elsevier; 2021. p. 206–12.
5. Renard D, Rubli E, Voide N, et al. Spectrum of digoxin-induced ocular toxicity: a case report and literature review. BMC Res Notes 2015;8:368.
6. Leong JK, Ghabrial R, Mccluskey PJ, et al. Orbital haemorrhage complication following postoperative thrombolysis. Br J Ophthalmol 2003;87(5):655–6.
7. Superstein R, Gomolin JE, Hammouda W, et al. Prevalence of ocular hemorrhage in patients receiving warfarin therapy. Can J Ophthalmol 2000;35(7):385–9.
8. Uyhazi KE, Miano T, Pan W, et al. Association of novel oral antithrombotics with the risk of intraocular bleeding. JAMA Ophthalmol 2018;136(2):122–30.
9. Shieh WS, Sridhar J, Hong BK, et al. Ophthalmic complications associated with direct oral anticoagulant medications. Semin Ophthalmol 2017;32(5):614–9.
10. Fraunfelder FT, Fraunfelder RW, editors. Drug-induced ocular side effects. 8th edition. New York: Elsevier; 2021. p. 100–7.
11. Erie JC, Brue SM, Chamberlain AM, et al. Selective serotonin reuptake inhibitor use and increased risk of cataract surgery: a population-based, case-control study. Am J Ophthalmol 2014;158(1):192–7. E1.
12. Fraunfelder FT, Fraunfelder RW, editors. Drug-induced ocular side effects. 8th edition. New York: Elsevier; 2021. p. 212–21.
13. Biaggioni I, Robertson D. Adrenoceptor agonists and sympathomimetic drugs. In: Basic and clinical pharmacology. 12th edition. San Francisco (CA): McGraw-Hill Medical; 2012. p. 151–5.
14. Abdel-Aziz S, Mamalis N. Intraoperative floppy iris syndrome. Curr Opin Ophthalmol 2009;20(1):37–41.
15. Zaman F, Bach C, Junaid I, et al. The floppy iris syndrome: what urologists and ophthalmologists need to know. Curr Urol 2012;6(1):1–7.

16. Aref A, Achiron A, Akkara J. Drug-induced acute angle closure glaucoma. 2019. Available at: https://eyewiki.aao.org/Drug-induced_Acute_Angle_Closure_ Glaucoma. Accessed August 23, 2020.

17. Burckhard BA, Ringeisen AL. Topical carbonic anhydrase inhibitors. In EyeWiki. April 15, 2020. Available at: https://eyewiki.org/Topical_Carbonic_ Anhydrase_ Inhibitors. Accessed September 1, 2020.

18. Jishi N, Adam M, Lee DW, et al. Central serous chorioretinopathy. In EyeWiki. 2020. Available at: https://eyewiki.org/Central_Serous_Chorioretinopathy. Accessed September 1, 2020.

19. Sambhara D, Vannadil H, Bracha P, et al. Sickle cell retinopathy. In EyeWiki. 2016. Available at: https://eyewiki.aao.org/Sickle_Cell_Retinopathy. Accessed September 30, 2020.

20. Ikeda N, Ikeda T, Nagata M, et al. Ciliochoroidal effusion syndrome induced by sulfa derivatives. Arch Ophthalmol 2002;120(12):1775.

21. Laties A, Sharlip I. Ocular safety in patients using sildenafil citrate therapy for erectile dysfunction. J Sex Med 2006;3(1):12–27.

22. Cordell WH, Maturi RK, Costigan TM, et al. Retinal effects of 6 months of daily use of tadalafil or sildenafil. Arch Ophthalmol 2009;127(4):367–73.

23. Miller NR, Arnold AC. Current concepts in the diagnosis, pathogenesis, and management of nonarteritic anterior ischemic optic neuropathy. Eye 2015;29:65–79.

24. Peponis V, Kyttaris VC, Chalkiadakis SE, et al. Ocular side effects of anti-rheumatic medications: what a rheumatologist should know. Lupus 2010;19(6): 675–82.

25. Ooi KG-J, Khoo P, Vaclavik V, et al. Statins in ophthalmology. Surv Ophthalmol 2019;64(3):401–32.

26. Tan NC, Yip WF, Kallakuri S, et al. Factors associated with impaired color vision without retinopathy amongst people with type 2 diabetes mellitus: a cross-sectional study. BMC Endocr Disord 2017;17(1):29.

27. Hampson JP, Harvey JN. A systematic review of drug induced ocular reactions in diabetes. Br J Ophthalmol 2000;84(2):144–9.

28. Keller JT. Second generation oral hypoglycemic agents. J Am Optom Assoc 1991;62(7):513–4.

29. Haug S, Wong R, Day S, et al. Didanosine retinal toxicity. Retina 2016;36(Suppl 1):S159–67.

30. Nguyen QD, Kempen JH, Bolton SG, et al. Immune recovery uveitis in patients with AIDS and cytomegalovirus retinitis after highly active antiretroviral therapy. Am J Ophthalmol 2000;129(5):634–9.

31. Stephenson M. Systemic drugs with ocular side effects. 2011. Available at: https://www.reviewofophthalmology.com/article/systemic-drugs-with-ocular-side-effects. Accessed September 22, 2020.

32. Saraiya N, Goldstein D. Drug-induced uveitis. 2020. Available at: https://eyewiki. aao.org/Drug_Induced_Uveitis#Bisphosphonates. Accessed September 25, 2020.

33. Mannino S, Troncon MG, Wallander M, et al. Ocular disorders in users of H2 antagonists and of omeprazole. Pharmacoepidemiol Drug Saf 1998;7:233–41.

34. Miller RD, Eriksson L, Fleisher LA, et al. Chapter 55, Airway management in the adult. In: Miller's anesthesia. 8th edition. Elsevier; 2015. p. 1647–81.

35. Katzung BG, Masters S. Basic & clinical pharmacology. San Francisco, CA: McGraw-Hill Medical; 2012.

36. Teo K, Yazdabadi A. Isotretinoin and night blindness. Australas J Dermatol 2014; 55(3):222–4.

37. Lee AG. Pseudotumor cerebri after treatment with tetracycline and isotretinoin for acne. Cutis 1995;55(3):165–8.
38. Roytman M, Frumkin A, Bohn TG. Pseudotumor cerebri caused by isotretinoin. Cutis 1988;42(5):399–400.
39. Rismondo V, Ubels JL. Isotretinoin in lacrimal gland fluid and tears. Arch Ophthalmol 1987;105(3):416–20.
40. Karimaghaei S, Karimaghaei C, Bindaganavile, et al. Ethambutol optic neuropathy. In: Eyewiki. 2020. Available at: https://eyewiki.org/Ethambutol_Optic_Neuropathy. Accessed September 1, 2020.
41. Kokkada S, Barthakur R, Natarajan, et al. Ocular side effects of antitubercular drugs - a focus on prevention, early detection and management. Kathmandu Univ Med J (Kumj) 2005;3:438–41.
42. Lan YW, Hsieh JW. Bilateral acute angle closure glaucoma and myopic shift by topiramate-induced ciliochoroidal effusion: case report and literature review. Int Ophthalmol 2018;38(6):2639–48.
43. Craig JE, Ong TJ, Louis DL, et al. Mechanism of topiramate-induced acute-onset myopia and angle closure glaucoma. Am J Ophthalmol 2004;137(1):193–5.
44. ELMIRON (pentosan polysulfate sodium) [Important Safety Information]. Titusville, NJ: Janssen Pharmaceuticals, Inc.; 2020.
45. Hanif AM, Armenti ST, Taylor SC, et al. Phenotypic spectrum of pentosan polysulfate sodium-associated maculopathy: a multicenter study. JAMA Ophthalmol 2019;137(11):1275–82.
46. Jain N, Bhatti T, Fekrat S. In. Eyenet. Macular edema associated with fingolimod. 2016. Available at: https://www.aao.org/eyenet/article/macular-edema-associated-with-fingolimod. Accessed September, 1, 2020.
47. Mandal P, Gupta A, Fusi-Rubiano W, et al. Fingolimod: therapeutic mechanisms and ocular adverse effects. Eye 2016;31(2):232–40.
48. Zarbin MA, Jampol LM, Jager RD, et al. Ophthalmic evaluations in clinical studies of fingolimod (FTY720) in multiple sclerosis. Ophthalmology 2013;120(7):1432–9.
49. Kim H-A, Lee S, Eah KS, et al. Prevalence and risk factors of tamoxifen retinopathy. Ophthalmology 2020;127(4):555–7.
50. Chhablani J, Zhu I, Lim JI, et al. Drug induced maculopathy. In: EyeWiki. 2020. Available at: https://eyewiki.org/Drug_induced_maculopathy. Accessed September 1, 2020.
51. Farkouh A, Frigo P, Czejka M. Systemic side effects of eye drops: a pharmacokinetic perspective. Clin Ophthalmol 2016;10:2433–41.
52. Kamjoo S, Barash A, Lim JI, et al. Intravitreal injections. In: EyeWiki. 2019. Available at: https://eyewiki.aao.org/Intravitreal_Injections. Accessed September 1, 2020.
53. Ortiz-Morales G, Garcia DL. Topical anesthetic abuse keratopathy. In: EyeWiki. 2020. Available at: https://eyewiki.org/Topical_Anesthetic_Abuse_Keratopathy. Accessed September 1, 2020.
54. Bakhsh S, Cheng O, Paro AM, et al. Comprehensive drop guide. In: EyeWiki. 2020. Available at: https://eyewiki.org/Comprehensive_Drop_Guide. Accessed September 1, 2020.

# Vision Restoration
## Cataract Surgery and Surgical Correction of Myopia, Hyperopia, and Presbyopia

Sonia H. Yoo, MD[a,b,*], Mike Zein, MD[c]

## KEYWORDS

- Cataract • Refractive surgery • Refractive error • Myopia • Presbyopia
- Astigmatism • Phacoemulsification • LASIK

## KEY POINTS

- The decision to remove the cataract rests mainly with the patient and planning for surgery is a combined effort between the patient, ophthalmologist, and primary care physician.
- More often than not, cataract surgery is also a refractive procedure with the potential of making the patient less spectacle-dependent for near, intermediate, and distance vision.
- Intraocular lens implants and surgical approaches continue to advance to allow each patient an individualized operative approach.
- Phacoemulsification remains the most common approach for cataract surgery around the world, with femtosecond laser–assisted cataract surgery emerging as a popular adjunct to phacoemulsification over the past decade.
- Refractive procedures, such as LASIK, SMILE, and PRK, are indicated for patients with refractive error in otherwise healthy eyes.

 Video content accompanies this article at http://www.medical.theclinics.com.

## INTRODUCTION

Advances in vision restoration procedures have developed over the past decade and have redefined what is considered possible for patients with refractive errors.[1] With

[a] Cornea and Refractive Surgery Department, Bascom Palmer Eye Institute, University of Miami Miller School of Medicine, 900 Northwest 17th Street, Miami, FL 33136, USA; [b] Department of Ophthalmology, Bascom Palmer Eye Institute, University of Miami Miller School of Medicine, 900 Northwest 17th Street, Miami, FL 33136, USA; [c] McKnight Vision Research Center, Bascom Palmer Eye Institute, University of Miami-Miller School of Medicine, 900 Northwest 17th Street, Miami, FL 33136, USA
* Corresponding author. Department of Ophthalmology, Bascom Palmer Eye Institute, University of Miami Miller School of Medicine, 900 Northwest 17th Street, Miami, FL 33136.
E-mail address: syoo@med.miami.edu

Med Clin N Am 105 (2021) 445–454
https://doi.org/10.1016/j.mcna.2021.01.002
0025-7125/21/© 2021 Elsevier Inc. All rights reserved.

cataract surgery being the most commonly performed surgical procedure in the United States and refractive surgery developing at a rapid pace, patient expectations for near perfect vision are unprecedented. Procedures, such as laser in situ keratomileusis (LASIK), photorefractive keratectomy (PRK), and small incision lenticule excision (SMILE), are continuously being improved to widen the eligibility criteria for patients. Correction of presbyopia, notoriously difficult to achieve, is now closer to realization than was considered possible.

Refractive surgical procedures entail altering the refractive components of the eye (the cornea and/or lens) to decrease or eliminate dependence on glasses and contact lenses. Corneal-based procedures are geared toward reshaping the surface of the cornea in patients with refractive errors (ametropia), and this is done by laser removal of corneal tissue from the surface (PRK), under a corneal flap (LASIK) or more recently, laser removal of corneal tissue through a corneal pocket (SMILE). These refractive procedures are indicated in healthy eyes without comorbid conditions. Lens-based procedures replace the natural crystalline lens with an artificial intraocular lens (IOL) implant. These procedures are indicated in patients with cataracts that diminish vision or make it difficult to visualize the retina. Another indication for lens removal is to prevent a particular type of glaucoma related to thickening of the lens. Less commonly, lens removal with an IOL implant is performed in the absence of a cataract for the sole purpose of reducing or eliminating the need for glasses. This is called a clear lens extraction. The type of procedure selected depends on the cause and degree of refractive error, patient's age, postoperative refractive target, type of cataract, and surgeon's experience.

## CATARACT
### Introduction

A cataract is defined as the opacification of a crystalline lens that over time can cause visual impairment in form of blurry vision, halos and glare around light, difficulty reading small print, and eventually blindness. Cataracts are classified as being age-related, secondary to systemic disease (ie, diabetes mellitus), secondary to primary ocular disease (uveitis, acute angle closure), traumatic, and congenital.

It is currently estimated that of the global population with moderate to severe vision impairment, 57.1 million cases are caused by cataract.[2] With an estimated 3.3 million procedures performed annually, cataract surgery is one of the most common procedures done in the United states. These projections are expected to increase to 4.4 million in 2030 as the US population continues to increase.[1]

### Causes and Associated Conditions

The development of cataracts occurs over time as part of the natural aging process of the lens. The crystalline protein that makes up more than 90% of the lens anatomy denatures and degrades with age, leading to a gradual opacification of the lens. Most patients do not develop visually significant cataracts until they are "very elderly," which is greater than or equal to 85 years old as defined by the World Health Organization and National Institute of aging.[3] The process is accelerated in patients with systemic conditions, such as diabetes, because of the high concentration of glucose in the aqueous humor diffusing into the lens. The glucose becomes metabolized into sorbitol and then results in osmotic overhydration, which leads to the development of opacities. Other systemic diseases that may result in cataract formation include myotonic dystrophy, atopic dermatitis, and neurofibromatosis type 2. Cataracts may also develop secondary to a primary ocular disease, including chronic anterior uveitis (secondary to prolonged inflammation and topical steroids the lens is exposed to), acute angle closure glaucoma (secondary to focal infarcts on the lens epithelium), high degrees of myopia (>-6 diopters), and congenital conditions (eg, hereditary retinal dystrophies).

Traumatic cataracts, as the name suggests, arise secondary to various forms of trauma and is the most common cause of unilateral cataracts in younger patients. Causes include penetrating, blunt, and radioactive trauma. In addition, these types of cataracts tend to be more challenging than the typical age-related cataracts because of a denser lens and weakened zonules, therefore increasing the risk for posterior dislocation of the lens intraoperatively.

## Indications for Surgery and Preoperative Evaluation

The most important factor to consider when assessing the suitability of a patient for cataract surgery is the impact of the cataract on the patient's ability to perform essential activities of daily living, such as driving, reading, and work involving near vision. Deciding when to remove the cataract rests mainly with the patient and their specific needs. In some cases, cataract surgery may be medically indicated when the cataract is adversely affecting the health of the eye, such as lens-induced glaucoma (phacolytic glaucoma).

Preoperative planning is a combined effort between the ophthalmologist and primary care physician. Because this is an elective procedure in most cases, a general medical history should be taken and the patient should be optimized with respect to their medical comorbidities (eg, diabetes, hypertension). This is more important if the patient requires general anesthesia, and preoperative assessment should be done as per local guidelines. In most cases, the procedure is done under monitored intravenous sedation with topical anesthetic and in some cases a local block is administered (retrobulbar, peribulbar, subconjunctival/subtenon). General anesthesia is considered in cases where the patient is uncooperative or experiencing severe anxiety surrounding the procedure.

It is also important to make note of the medications that the patient is taking at the time of referral/consultation. Relevant medications include systemic α-blockers (eg, tamsulosin), which can lead to intraoperative floppy iris syndrome, the triad of iris billowing, pupil constriction, and iris prolapse. Intraoperative floppy iris syndrome may make the procedure more difficult and necessitate the need for iris retractors. The literature suggests that in patients who have a history of systemic α-blockers use, discontinuation preoperatively has little to no effect in mitigating intraoperative floppy iris syndrome; however, it is still important for the surgeon to be aware before the procedure to adequately prepare for the surgery.[4] With respect to anticoagulant and antiplatelet therapy, management should be as per local protocols. Although most surgeons do not stop these medications preoperatively, the international normalized ratio should be within therapeutic range 24 hours before surgery in otherwise stable patients. When possible, some surgeons do prefer to stop aspirin a week to 10 days before surgery. Cataract surgery is considered a low-risk operation for bleeding. Modifying certain surgical details (eg, the use of topical anesthesia rather than retrobulbar block or the use of intraoperative mydriatic rather than iris retractors) is done to further reduce bleeding risk in this group of patients.

In terms of the ophthalmic preoperative assessment, biometry plays an essential role in the planning of a successful procedure with satisfactory visual and refractive outcomes. Keratometry and biometry, defined next, are needed to calculate the IOL power for the patient.

- *Keratometry*: Done to determine the anterior corneal surface curvature. This is defined as diopters or millimeters of radius of curvature. This is assessed by a keratometer or by corneal topography.
- *Optical coherence biometry*: Measures the axial length (the total length of the eye) through a noncontact method that uses two coaxial partially coherent low-energy laser beams to procedure an interference pattern.
- *IOL power calculation*: Various formulae exists that are used to calculate the required IOL power needed to achieve the desired refractive outcome.

### Intraocular Lens Options

The first IOL was implanted in 1949, and their use in cataract surgery has become standard since the 1970s.[5] With advances in cataract surgery, such as the introduction of phacoemulsification allowing for smaller corneal incisions, shorter postoperative recovery periods, and more pliable IOLs, a myriad of options now exist tailored to the visual goals of the patient. The choice of IOL is determined by the patient's visual preferences, type and degree of astigmatism, and refractive error.

- Monofocal IOLs
  - These are by far the most common option for IOL implants in cataract surgery. Monofocal IOLs are geared toward improving the patient's uncorrected visual acuity at a single focal point (near, intermediate, or distance vision). This option still requires the use of glasses postoperatively either for distance or near, or sometimes both. A common scenario is a patient who has cataracts and opts for a monofocal lens in both eyes to correct them for distance vision without glasses. The patient would then require glasses to wear for near activities. The exception is for patients with planned "monovision" where one eye is targeted for distance and the other eye for near. This allows for less dependence on glasses postoperatively, but may not be tolerated by all patients and requires careful patient selection (**Fig. 1A**).
- Multifocal and extended depth of focus IOLs
  - Unlike monofocal IOLs, multifocal and extended depth of focus IOLs offer the benefit of potential spectacle independence. In multifocal lenses, the expanded range of vision is because of the added magnification in different zones or rings of the lens allowing the patient to see at near, intermediate, and distance. In extended depth of focus lenses, there is a single elongated focal point to enhance the depth of focus. The drawbacks of multifocal and extended depth of focus lenses include the increased likelihood of glare and haloes especially at night (**Fig. 1B**).
- Toric IOLs
  - Toric IOLs are considered in patients with astigmatism in addition to a cataract. The toric IOL is suitable for patients with astigmatism because of the lens having different powers in different meridians allowing for the surgeon to adjust the orientation of the IOL based on the patient's degree of astigmatism.
  - Toric IOLs have to a large extent decreased the need for limbal-relaxing incisions intraoperatively. These are small incisions made at opposite ends of the cornea at the junction between the cornea and sclera (the limbus), to alter the curvature of the cornea making it more spherical in shape. This is done in cases of low to moderate astigmatism, and is sometimes performed with a femtosecond laser instead of toric IOL placement.
  - Patients may require further refractive surgery (eg, LASIK, PRK) after toric IOL placement in the event of residual astigmatism (**Fig. 2**).

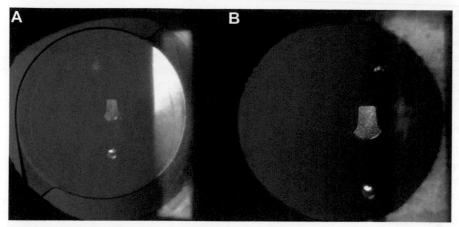

Fig. 1. (A) Monofocal IOL. (B) Multifocal IOL.

- Accommodative IOLs
  - Like the multifocal IOLs, the accommodative IOL offers the option of spectacle independence. This IOL is unique in design compared with other alternatives by virtue of its aspheric shape and flexible haptics. As the name suggests, the flexible haptics allow for accommodation whereby they slightly move the IOL forward when using near vision. The trade-off, however, is in a reduced level of magnification compared with a multifocal IOL. Studies have shown multifocal IOLs to be superior to accommodative IOLs with respect to near vision.[6,7]

## SURGICAL TECHNIQUES

Cataract surgery has evolved significantly over the past two millennia, from its ancient and crude predecessor "couching" in the fifth century, to the more sophisticated techniques of today.[8] The first recorded cataract removal was performed in Paris in 1748.[9,10] Since its invention in 1967, phacoemulsification has become the most popular cataract removal technique in the developed world.[5] Since its Food and Drug

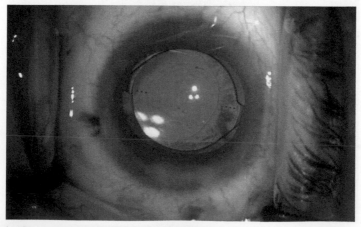

Fig. 2. Toric IOL.

Administration approval in 2010, femtosecond laser–assisted cataract surgery has been gaining popularity as an adjunct to phacoemulsification, especially for patients with astigmatism. The preferred choice of technique depends on surgeon discretion and opinions differ among surgeons regarding the safety, complication rate, and cost-effectiveness of the two options. Ultimately, the patient's preferences, refractive goal, choice of IOLs, whether the patient has astigmatism, and the density of the cataract figure into the decision about which technique is best for the patient.

### Phacoemulsification

The traditional approach, phacoemulsification, is the most commonly performed cataract surgery worldwide and is performed by the breakdown of the crystalline lens into small enough fragments, by ultrasound energy, which are aspirated out of the anterior chamber through a phacoemulsification tip handpiece.

### Surgical steps

1. Topical proparacaine or tetracaine drops are applied followed by povidone-iodine 5% into the conjunctival sac. Ophthalmic lidocaine gel then is instilled onto the ocular surface. Eyelids and eyelashes are cleaned thoroughly. Antiseptic is left in place to have its affect for 3 minutes followed by an eye rinse with sterile saline.
   * Consider retrobulbar or peribulbar injection, intravenous sedation or general anesthesia if there is concern over patient's ability to cooperate during procedure.
2. A side port incision is made approximately 60° left of main incision (**Fig. 3**).
3. Viscoelastic is injected into the anterior chamber (Video 1).

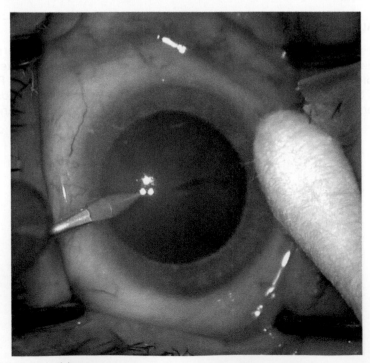

**Fig. 3.** Side port incision.

4. A main corneal or perilimbal incision is made with a keratome.
5. A continuous curvilinear capsulorhexis is performed, whereby a tear is created in the capsule and then guided in a continuous and curvilinear fashion around the anterior surface of the lens capsule (Video 2).
6. Nuclear disassembly is performed by first undergoing hydrodissection and hydro-delineation, the process of separating the nucleus and cortex of the lens from the capsule. This allows for manipulation of the nucleus for disassembly with the phacoemulsification handpiece (Video 3).
7. Aspiration of lens cortex is done carefully via vacuum (Video 4). This step is essential to mitigate postoperative inflammation and allow for optimal centration of IOL implant. Extra care must be taken when aspirating; it should be done slowly so as to monitor for any wrinkles in posterior capsule, which may indicate engagement of the posterior capsule.
8. IOL implantation is initiated by filling of the capsular bag with viscoelastic, followed by the introduction of a loaded injector cartridge with the IOL slowly injected and unrolled inside the capsular bag (Video 5). When using a toric IOL it is important to carefully observe while rotating the IOL to ensure that the haptics are within the capsular bag and that the optic is correctly aligned. Once the surgeon is satisfied with the positioning of the IOL, the viscoelastic should be aspirated to reduce the risk of postoperative rise in intraocular pressure.
9. Incisions are closed by hydrosealing (stromal saline injection). In some cases, the incisions may be closed by suturing. The surgeon may adopt several prophylactic measures to prevent postoperative endophthalmitis, such as intracameral, subconjunctival, or topical antibiotics with or without the use of steroids.

### Femtosecond Laser–Assisted Cataract Surgery

The use of femtosecond laser technology in cataract surgery has steadily gained popularity over the past decade. The femtosecond laser is able to perform four of the steps related to cataract surgery: (1) the corneal incisions (main incision and side ports), (2) incisions into the peripheral cornea to reduce astigmatism, (3) the capsulorhexis, and (4) the initial fragmentation of the crystalline lens. The remainder of the procedure is continued manually, which includes the phacoemulsification of the lens and aspiration of lens cortex.

The advantages to this approach include better circularity and centration of the capsulorhexis to allow for more precise positioning of the IOL and reduced expenditure of ultrasonic energy when removing lens fragments. It often is offered to patients with astigmatism.

Disadvantages to this approach include the higher out-of-pocket costs to the patient compared with standard phacoemulsification, the steep learning curve, longer total operating times, and perceived difficulty with certain complex cases (eg, small pupils).

### How Much Will it Cost?

Because cataract surgery is a medically necessary procedure, most of the costs associated with cataract surgery are covered by health insurance. The standard cost includes removal of the cataract, standard monofocal IOL, and may cover either a set of prescription glasses or contact lenses after the procedure. Decreasing dependence on glasses or contact lenses is not considered a medical necessity and therefore, the addition of premium IOLs to reduce such dependence and the addition of femtosecond laser technology to treat astigmatism are typically services not covered by insurance.

## Complications

Cataract surgery, like any operative procedure, comes with risks of infection and bleeding. The main ones specific to ocular surgery to be aware of include the following:

- *Endophthalmitis*: This is defined as an acute (within 4 weeks of surgery) or chronic (>4 weeks after surgery) inflammation of the internal content (tissue or fluid) of the eye secondary to an infection. Symptoms include pain, redness, and vision loss, with inflammatory signs of conjunctival injection, and/or hypopyon. Sometimes the source of infection is hard to identify with complete certainty but it is thought to be from the resident flora of conjunctiva and eyelids. Possible risk factors include posterior lens capsule rupture during surgery, prolonged procedure time, and delay in receiving postoperative antibiotics. Evidence has shown that administering intracameral antibiotics into the anterior chamber at the end of the procedure may reduce the risk of endophthalmitis.[11] However, the use of intracameral antibiotics is still controversial in the United States and has not been universally adopted. Thankfully, this is a rare complication with an incidence around 0.1% in contemporary literature.[12,13]
- *Posterior capsular opacification*: With a varied incidence in the literature of 5% to 50%, this is the most common delayed onset finding of an otherwise uncomplicated cataract surgery.[14–16] Posterior capsular opacification is also referred to as an "after cataract" and occurs because of the proliferation and migration of lens epithelial cells. It is universally seen in children after cataract surgery. Posterior capsular opacification is straightforward to treat in the clinic setting. This is done by performing a posterior capsulotomy with a neodymium:yttrium-aluminum-garnet laser (**Fig. 4**).

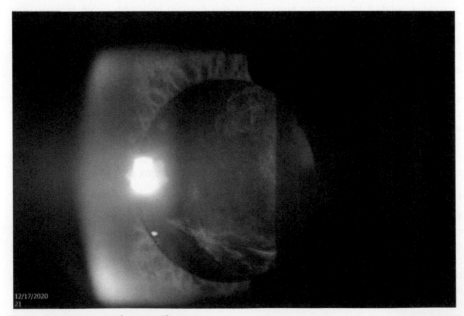

**Fig. 4.** Posterior capsular opacification.

### Refractive Procedures

Although cataract surgery is a form of refractive surgery, other options exists for patients with otherwise healthy eyes that do not have an opacified lens obscuring vision. These options include LASIK, SMILE, and PRK. These procedures improve the patient's vision by reshaping the surface of the eye, the cornea, by either an excimer laser, a femtosecond laser, or both depending on the procedure chosen. LASIK is the most common of the previously mentioned procedures and is defined by its superb visual outcomes, quick postoperative recovery periods, and minimal risk of complications.

## DISCUSSION
### Future Directions

The continuing advances in IOL technologies in the form of EDF IOLs, low-add multifocals, trifocals, and adjustable IOL technology do not seem to be slowing down. The current market penetration of presbyopic IOLs is around 8%, and with surgeons becoming more confident they can achieve a patient's desired refractive outcome and the continual improvement of technology, that figure will only rise. In addition, fewer patients may require corneal refractive surgery as surgeons achieve improved refractive outcomes with cataract refractive surgery. Furthermore, the holy grail that is the correction of presbyopia may be closer to reality than a dream with advancements in IOL technology and development of drugs allowing for true restoration of accommodation.

## SUMMARY

Vision restoration procedures continue to advance at a rapid pace with exceptional outcomes. It is important to remember that cataract surgery is a form of refractive surgery. Many patients who previously could not contemplate being independent of glasses or contact lenses can now select from a myriad of surgical approaches and premium IOLs. With the development of improved biometry and lens formulae to aid in hitting the refractive target, to the advancement of premium IOL designs and femtosecond laser–assisted procedures, the horizon for further advances in cataract and refractive surgery bodes well.

## CLINICS CARE POINTS

- The standard IOL used in cataract surgery is the monofocal lens; however, premium upgrades include the multifocal lens for presbyopia and the femtosecond laser and toric lens for astigmatism.

- Detailed history of patients' medications and comorbidities is essential for preoperative planning and assessment; patients on $\alpha$-blockers are predisposed to floppy iris syndrome, which may necessitate the need for iris retractors.

- Anticoagulation and antiplatelet therapy may be continued if medically necessary because cataract surgery is considered a low-risk operation for bleeding. However, communication between the ophthalmologist and primary care physician/internist is important because certain surgical details are modified to further lower the risk of bleeding for patients on these types of medications.

- Endophthalmitis is one of most serious complications associated with cataract surgery; however, it is rare with an incidence of less than 0.1%.

## ACKNOWLEDGEMENT

Grant: Supported by NIH Center Core Grant P30EY014801, Research to Prevent Blindness Unrestricted Grant.

## DISCLOSURE

The authors have no relevant disclosures.

## SUPPLEMENTARY DATA

Supplementary data related to this article can be found online at https://doi.org/10.1016/j.mcna.2021.01.002.

## REFERENCES

1. Schein OD, Cassard SD, Tielsch JM, et al. Cataract surgery among Medicare beneficiaries. Ophthalmic Epidemiol 2012;19(5):257–64.
2. Flaxman SR, Bourne RRA, Resnikoff S, et al. Global causes of blindness and distance vision impairment 1990-2020: a systematic review and meta-analysis. Lancet Glob Health 2017;5(12):e1221–34.
3. Olson RJ, Braga-Mele R, Chen SH, et al. Cataract in the adult eye preferred practice pattern. Ophthalmology 2017;124(2):P1–119.
4. Chang DF, Braga-Mele R, Mamalis N, et al. ASCRS White Paper: clinical review of intraoperative floppy-iris syndrome. J Cataract Refract Surg 2008;34(12): 2153–62.
5. Davis G. The evolution of cataract surgery. Mo Med 2016;113(1):58–62.
6. Tan N, Zheng D, Ye J. Comparison of visual performance after implantation of 3 types of intraocular lenses: accommodative, multifocal, and monofocal. Eur J Ophthalmol 2014;24(5):693–8.
7. Lan J, Huang YS, Dai YH, et al. Visual performance with accommodating and multifocal intraocular lenses. Int J Ophthalmol 2017;10(2):235–40.
8. Aruta A, Marenco M, Marinozzi S. [History of cataract surgery]. Med Secoli 2009; 21(1):403–28.
9. Daviel J. Lettre sur les maladies des yeux. Paris: Mercure de France; 1748. p. 1748.
10. Rucker CW. Cataract: a historical perspective. Invest Ophthalmol 1965;4:377–83.
11. Gower EW, Lindsley K, Tulenko SE, et al. Perioperative antibiotics for prevention of acute endophthalmitis after cataract surgery. Cochrane Database Syst Rev 2017;2(2):CD006364.
12. Astley RA, Coburn PS, Parkunan SM, et al. Modeling intraocular bacterial infections. Prog Retin Eye Res 2016;54:30–48.
13. Durand ML. Bacterial and fungal endophthalmitis. Clin Microbiol Rev 2017;30(3): 597–613.
14. Schmidbauer JM, Vargas LG, Apple DJ, et al. Evaluation of neodymium:yttrium-aluminum-garnet capsulotomies in eyes implanted with AcrySof intraocular lenses. Ophthalmology 2002;109(8):1421–6.
15. Dholakia SA, Vasavada AR. Intraoperative performance and longterm outcome of phacoemulsification in age-related cataract. Indian J Ophthalmol 2004;52(4): 311–7.
16. Thompson AM, Sachdev N, Wong T, et al. The Auckland Cataract Study: 2 year postoperative assessment of aspects of clinical, visual, corneal topographic and satisfaction outcomes. Br J Ophthalmol 2004;88(8):1042–8.

# Diabetic and Retinal Vascular Eye Disease

Hong-Gam Le, MD*, Akbar Shakoor, MD

## KEYWORDS

- Diabetic retinopathy • Diabetic macular edema • Retinal vascular disease
- Retinal vein occlusion • Retinal artery occlusion

## KEY POINTS

- Diabetic retinopathy is the leading cause of blindness in working-age adults.
- Blood glucose and blood pressure control can lower the risk of diabetic retinopathy.
- Routine dilated ophthalmologic examinations can aid in earlier recognition and treatment of diabetic retinopathy and reduce the risk of vision loss. Telemedicine can facilitate easier access to diabetic retinopathy screening.
- Retinal vein occlusion in patients younger than age 50 and in those without known vascular risk factors should prompt further workup for underlying systemic disorders.
- Patients presenting with acute painless vision loss concerning for retinal artery occlusion require emergent stroke workup.

## DIABETIC RETINOPATHY
### How Common Is Diabetic Retinopathy?

Diabetic retinopathy, a microvascular complication of diabetes mellitus, is the leading cause of blindness worldwide among patients aged 25 to 75.[1] It occurs in both type 1 and type 2 diabetes. Diabetes affected 463 million people in 2019, and its prevalence is expected to increase to 700 million by 2040.[2] About one-third of patients with diabetes have diabetic retinopathy, and 1 in 10 patients will develop vision-threatening disease.[3,4] In the United States alone, approximately 1 in 10 people have diabetes.[5] In 2010, approximately 7.7 million Americans had diabetic retinopathy, and this number is projected to double to 14.6 million by 2050.[6]

The prevalence of diabetic retinopathy increases with the duration of diabetes. After 20 years of living with diabetes, approximately 99% of patients with type 1 diabetes and 60% of patients with type 2 diabetes develop some form of diabetic retinopathy.[7]

The Diabetes Control and Complications Trial (DCCT)[8] and United Kingdom Prospective Diabetes Study (UKPDS),[9] both randomized clinical trials, have shown that intensive glycemic control reduces diabetic complications, including retinopathy, in both type 1 and type 2 diabetes.

John A. Moran Eye Center, 65 North Mario Capecchi Drive, Salt Lake City, UT 84132, USA
* Corresponding author.
*E-mail addresses:* hong-gam.le@hsc.utah.edu; hgle888@gmail.com

Med Clin N Am 105 (2021) 455–472
https://doi.org/10.1016/j.mcna.2021.02.004
0025-7125/21/© 2021 Elsevier Inc. All rights reserved.

## How Does Diabetes Cause Damage to the Retina?

Diabetic retinopathy occurs because of damage to retinal capillaries caused by prolonged exposure to hyperglycemia.[10] Although not yet well-delineated, the pathophysiology is thought to involve several biochemical reactions, including increases in inflammatory oxidative stress, advanced glycation end products, and protein kinase C pathways. The net effect results in endothelial damage, basement membrane thickening, and pericyte loss. Over time, damage to retinal capillaries leads to capillary occlusion and retinal ischemia. In addition, the compromised endothelial barrier leads to serum leakage and retinal edema. In late-stage retinopathy, ischemic retinal tissue produces intraocular vascular endothelial growth factor (VEGF), which promotes intraocular neovascularization. These abnormal blood vessels are fragile and can bleed within the eye, causing vision loss and elevated intraocular pressure. When regressed, the fibrotic neovascular remnants can exert traction on the retina, leading to retinal detachment.

## How Is Diabetic Retinopathy Staged?

Diabetic retinopathy is staged on a severity scale based on clinical features seen on dilated fundus examination.[11] Ophthalmologists first classify disease as either nonproliferative diabetic retinopathy (NPDR) or proliferative diabetic retinopathy (PDR). The key difference between NPDR and PDR is the presence of neovascularization in PDR.

NPDR is graded as mild, moderate, severe, or very severe depending on the observed intraretinal pathology, including microaneurysms, intraretinal hemorrhages, venous beading, and intraretinal microvascular abnormalities (**Fig. 1**). Proliferative diabetic retinopathy is graded non-high-risk versus high-risk. Non-high-risk PDR may have mild neovascularization of the optic nerve head and/or neovascularization elsewhere in the retina but does not have vitreous hemorrhage (**Fig. 2**). High-risk PDR is characterized by moderate to severe neovascularization of the optic nerve head or neovascularization elsewhere in the retina with vitreous hemorrhage (**Fig. 3**). Diabetic macular edema (DME), which is swelling of the central retina, may occur at any stage of retinopathy. Proper documentation of a diabetic eye examination requires both grading of retinopathy and description of DME.

Higher levels of glycosylated hemoglobin (HbA1c) correlate with the progression of retinopathy from mild NPDR to high-risk PDR.[12] Patients with severe NPDR have a 15% risk of progression to high-risk PDR within 1 year. The risk is increased to

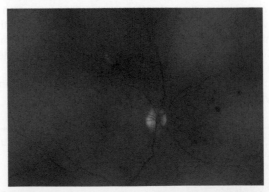

**Fig. 1.** Severe NPDR. Fundus photograph of the right eye shows diffuse microaneurysms and intraretinal hemorrhages in all 4 quadrants.

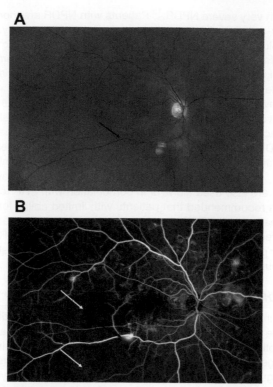

**Fig. 2.** Non-high-risk PDR. (*A*) Fundus photograph of the right eye shows a net of neovascularization along the inferior vascular arcade (*black arrow*). (*B*) Fluorescein angiogram demonstrates neovascularization and areas of nonperfusion (*yellow arrows*). Note that there is no neovascularization of the optic nerve head and no vitreous hemorrhage.

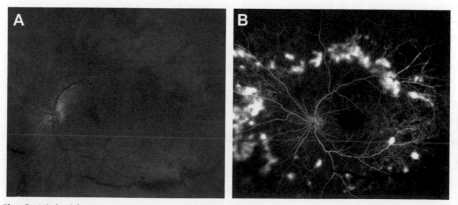

**Fig. 3.** High-risk PDR with vitreous hemorrhage. (*A*) Fundus photograph of the left eye shows neovascularization along the superior vascular arcade and vitreous hemorrhage settling inferiorly. (*B*) Fluorescein angiogram reveals more extensive neovascularization and multiple areas of non-perfusion.

45% for those with very severe NPDR.[13] Patients with NPDR are therefore monitored at different follow-up intervals depending on their disease severity. No ophthalmic treatment is absolutely indicated unless visually significant diabetic macular edema is present. Patients should be educated on the importance of systemic management including blood glucose and blood pressure control to lower the risk of retinopathy progression.[14] The DCCT showed that intensive glycemic control reduced the risk by 34% to 76% over the entire spectrum of retinopathy, thereby reducing the need for laser treatment and loss of vision.[8,15] Tight glycemic control remains the most critical and most effective strategy for preventing vision loss from diabetic retinopathy.

Patients with PDR, especially those with high-risk features, are treated with panretinal photocoagulation (PRP).[16] This treatment destroys the ischemic retina to minimize production of VEGF, thereby preventing neovascularization. Intravitreal anti-VEGF agents are also used alone or in combination with PRP to control neovascularization.[17] It is recommended that patients with limited ability for close follow-up receive PRP instead of anti-VEGF monotherapy, as the latter is shorter-acting, more costly, and requires repeated treatments for effect. Prophylactic PRP has also been recommended for patients with very severe NPDR who are at high risk for progression and/or have difficulty with routine follow-up.[13]

### When and How Often Should Patients with Diabetes Be Screened?

Screening recommendations vary depending on the types of diabetes, and on whether or not the patient is pregnant (**Table 1**).[11] Diabetic retinopathy is rare within the first 5 years following the diagnosis of type 1 diabetes mellitus. In contrast, a significant percentage of patients with type 2 diabetes already have retinopathy at the time of initial diagnosis. The recommended time of first dilated eye examination is thus 5 years after diagnosis for patients with type 1 diabetes, and immediately at diagnosis for patients with type 2 diabetes. Pregnancy increases the risk of progression of diabetic retinopathy—thus, pregnant women with any type of diabetes should have a dilated eye examination early in the first trimester and frequent follow-up. According to the Diabetes Report Card 2017, the dilated eye examination is one of the key preventative care practices that help patients better manage their condition and improve their health.[18] Several level 1, randomized, controlled studies[13,16,19] demonstrate the effectiveness of timely treatment in reducing the rate and severity of vision loss from diabetic retinopathy. It is therefore critical that patients with diabetes receive routine dilated eye examinations, which are necessary to detect complications of diabetic retinopathy.

Over the past decade, the use of nonmydriatic cameras for retinal imaging, combined with the remote evaluation of images at a telemedicine reading center, has

**Table 1**
**Dilated eye examination schedule for patients with diabetes mellitus**

| Diabetes Type | Initial Evaluation | Follow-up |
|---|---|---|
| Type 1 | 5 years after diagnosis | Annually |
| Type 2 | At time of diagnosis | Annually |
| Pregnancy with type 1 or type 2 | Soon after conception and early in the first trimester | Every 3 months |

*Modified from* American Academy of Ophthalmology Retina/Vitreous Panel. Preferred Practice Pattern® Guidelines. Diabetic Retinopathy. San Francisco: American Academy of Ophthalmology; 2019. Available at www.aao.org/ppp.

been utilized for diabetic retinopathy screening.[20] Such strategies implemented in primary care settings have been shown to increase screening rates among patients with diabetes, including those who are at high risk of missing recommended eye examinations.[21,22] Currently, an estimated one-third of adults with diabetes in the United States do not receive an annual dilated eye examination. Because most patients with diabetes have regular contact with primary care physicians, telemedicine screening in primary care and/or a medical subspecialist's office has immense potential to provide convenient and timely diabetic retinopathy screening to many patients.[23] Telemedicine diabetic retinopathy screening programs also have the collateral benefit of detecting other ocular conditions including cataract, hypertensive retinopathy, glaucoma, and age-related macular degeneration.[20]

### When and How Often Should Patients with Diabetic Retinopathy See a Retina Specialist?

An optometrist or a general ophthalmologist can perform the initial screening examination. Depending on the severity of disease, the patient may then be referred to a retina specialist for further evaluation. In addition to a dilated fundus examination, patients may undergo ancillary studies including optical coherence tomography (OCT) imaging and fluorescein angiogram (FA) to better evaluate the retinopathy. The follow-up interval is dictated by the disease severity and by the presence and type of DME, which can occur at any stage of retinopathy (**Table 2**).[11] Nonpregnant patients with diabetes should have a dilated eye examination at least once per year and as often as every 1 to 6 months depending on disease severity. Patients with DME affecting the center of their vision, for example, may even require monthly evaluation for intravitreal injections. In general, any patient with proliferative diabetic retinopathy and/or visually significant diabetic macular edema requires the care of a retinal specialist.

**Table 2**
**Dilated eye examination schedule for patients with diabetic retinopathy with or without diabetic macular edema**

| Diabetic Retinopathy Severity | Follow-up (months) | | |
| --- | --- | --- | --- |
| | No DME | NCI DME | CI DME |
| Mild NPDR | 12 | 4–6 | 1 |
| Moderate NPDR | 6–12 | 3–6 | 1 |
| Severe NPDR | 4 | 2–4 | 1 |
| PDR | 4 | 2–4 | 1 |

*Abbreviations:* CI DME, center-involved diabetic macular edema; DME, diabetic macular edema; NCI DME, non– center-involved diabetic macular edema; NPDR, nonproliferative diabetic retinopathy; PDR, proliferative diabetic retinopathy.
*Modified from* American Academy of Ophthalmology Retina/Vitreous Panel. Preferred Practice Pattern® Guidelines. Diabetic Retinopathy. San Francisco: American Academy of Ophthalmology; 2019. Available at www.aao.org/ppp.

### How Does Diabetic Retinopathy Cause Vision Loss?

In the early stages of diabetic retinopathy, especially in the absence of macular edema, patients are often asymptomatic. In the late stages, it is common for patients with poorly controlled diabetes to present with devastating vision loss caused by different manifestations of the disease.

Patients with diabetic retinopathy can develop acute, subacute, or chronic vision loss by several mechanisms:

- Capillary leakage → diabetic macular edema
- Capillary occlusion → macular ischemia → macular atrophy
- Sequela of ischemia-induced neovascularization, including vitreous hemorrhage, tractional retinal detachment, and neovascular glaucoma

Capillary leakage causes diabetic macular edema. Capillary occlusion involving the central retina can lead to ischemic maculopathy. Longstanding and severe disease can lead to vision-threatening conditions including macular atrophy and complications from ischemia-induced neovascularization: vitreous hemorrhage, tractional retinal detachment, and neovascular glaucoma.

### Diabetic macular edema

DME is caused by capillary leakage in the setting of a decompensated endothelial barrier of the retinal vasculature. Higher HbA1c levels are associated with increased risk of developing and progressing DME.[24] Poorly controlled hypertension also contributes to worsening of DME.[9]

DME can occur at any stage of diabetic retinopathy and is classified based on whether or not the edema involves the center of the retina (the fovea) as seen on OCT imaging (**Fig. 4**). Center-involved (CI-DME) portends a worse prognosis compared with non-centered-involved DME (NCI-DME), as the risk of visual loss is greater if the swelling is at the fovea. Thus, patients with CI-DME are recommended to have more frequent follow-up.

It is important to note, however, that the amount of edema does not always correlate with the degree of vision loss. Many patients can be asymptomatic with good visual

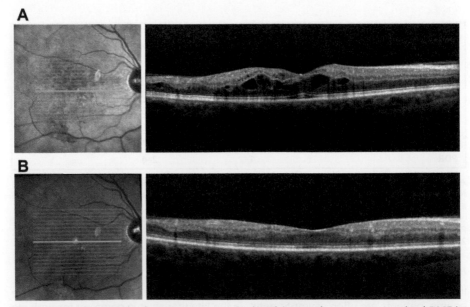

**Fig. 4.** DME. (*A*) Optical coherence tomography (OCT) image shows center-involved DME in the right eye. (*B*) Resolution of DME after treatment with intravitreal aflibercept (Eylea) in the same eye.

acuity despite the presence of CI-DME. Education on blood sugar control and close monitoring is appropriate for these patients.

Patients with visually significant DME can be treated with intravitreal anti-VEGF, intravitreal corticosteroids, and/or focal laser photocoagulation. Intravitreal anti-VEGF agents are currently the first line therapy, and include bevacizumab (Avastin), aflibercept (Eylea), and ranibizumab (Lucentis).[25] Of note, glitazone class of oral anti-hyperglycemic agents such as rosiglitazone and pioglitazone should be used with caution in patients with DME, as these agents have been associated with development or worsening of macular edema.[26]

### Ischemic maculopathy
Hyperglycemia-induced microvascular damages lead to retinal capillary occlusion and retinal ischemia. If this occurs in the central retina, patients develop gradual and permanent vision loss. Although other causes of vision loss in diabetic eyes such as macular edema, vitreous hemorrhage, or retinal detachment can be seen on dilated fundus examination, the diagnosis of macular ischemia often requires ophthalmic imaging.[27] Macular ischemia can be visualized on OCT angiogram or fluorescein angiogram as an enlarged foveal avascular zone (**Fig. 5**). Over time, an ischemic macula can become atrophic. On OCT, the retina appears thin with loss of photoreceptors and attenuation of retinal layers (**Fig. 6**).

### Vitreous hemorrhage
Vitreous hemorrhage is a potential complication of proliferative diabetic retinopathy characterized by intraocular bleeding within the vitreous cavity (**Fig. 7**). The up-regulation of VEGF induced by retinal ischemia leads to the growth of abnormal blood vessels. These vessels are friable and prone to spontaneous bleeding. Patients may present with symptoms ranging from mild blurry vision to sudden, severe vision loss. Patients also frequently describe increased floaters, a hazy hue in vision, or dark strands in their field of vision. These symptoms are caused by the diffuse red blood cells or blood clots that adhere to vitreous strands. Diabetic retinopathy is the most common underlying etiology in adults presenting with vitreous hemorrhage.

When a patient presents with vitreous hemorrhage, the most important first step of the management is to rule out the presence of retinal tear and/or retinal detachment. If the vitreous hemorrhage is severe enough to obscure the view to the retina, then

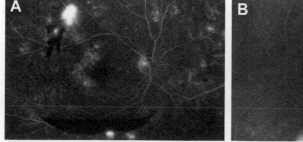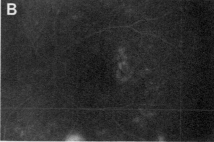

**Fig. 5.** Macular ischemia. (*A*) Fluorescein angiogram of the right eye with proliferative diabetic retinopathy demonstrates capillary nonperfusion in the center of the macula and thus an enlarged foveal avascular zone compared to that of the contralateral eye of the same patient. There is also capillary leakage, neovascularization, and preretinal hemorrhage. (*B*) Fluorescein angiogram of the left eye is notable for microaneurysms, capillary leakage, and neovascularization.

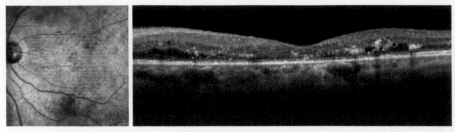

**Fig. 6.** Macular atrophy. Optical coherence tomography (OCT) image of the left eye shows central thinning of the retina and attenuation of the outer retinal layers.

ocular ultrasound is indicated to rule out retinal detachment. Immediate treatment options include anti-VEGF and/or laser photocoagulation if possible. Importantly, vitreous hemorrhage is not a contraindication to continuing systemic anticoagulant medications (such as aspirin, clopidogrel, or coumadin) that are indicated for other medical reasons.[28] Patients should avoid nonsteroidal anti-inflammatory drugs (NSAIDs) such as ibuprofen if possible. Pars plana vitrectomy with endolaser is the treatment for nonclearing vitreous hemorrhage. Early surgical intervention has been shown to improve visual outcomes in patients with type 1 diabetes, but not type 2 diabetes.[29]

### Retinal detachment

Patients with proliferative diabetic retinopathy are also at increased risk of vision loss from retinal detachment. When retinal neovascularization extends into the vitreous and proliferates into fibrovascular tissues, the resulting traction can cause retinal detachment (**Fig. 8**). If this complication occurs outside of the macula, the patient may remain asymptomatic for many years. If retinal detachment involves or threatens the macula, patients will develop vision loss and may describe photopsia because of traction exerted on the retina. Prompt surgical intervention with vitrectomy and removal of proliferative tissues is then indicated. Contraction of the fibrovascular tissues may cause a retinal break, leading to a combined tractional and rhegmatogenous

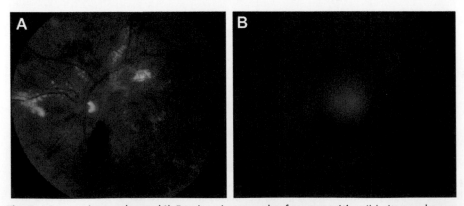

**Fig. 7.** Vitreous hemorrhage. (*A*) Fundus photograph of an eye with mild vitreous hemorrhage, most of which has settled inferiorly. There is sufficient view to deliver laser photocoagulation in areas of the retina not obscured by blood. (*B*) Fundus photograph of a different eye with diffuse vitreous hemorrhage limiting visualization of the entire retina.

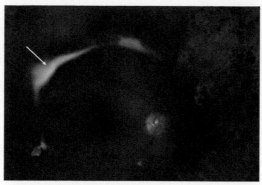

**Fig. 8.** Retinal detachment. Fundus photograph of the right eye shows fibrotic tissue (*arrow*) causing tractional retinal detachment that is threatening the macula.

retinal detachment. Urgent or emergent surgery is recommended for these patients. Patients frequently require placement of expansile gas or silicone oil in the eye as part of the operation. After surgery, patients are instructed to adhere to a certain position to optimize the chance of retina reattachment. If expansile gas is used, patients will be restricted from flying in airplanes or traveling over areas of high elevation such as mountains until the gas bubble is resorbed, which may take 3 to 8 weeks.[30] The use of nitrous oxide anesthesia in patients with intraocular gas is contraindicated as the mixture of gas and nitrous oxide can cause irreversible vision loss.[31]

### Neovascular glaucoma

In the proliferative stage of diabetic retinopathy, neovascularization can also result in abnormal vessel growth on the iris and within the angle of the anterior chamber, leading to a form of angle closure glaucoma.[11] Patients with neovascular glaucoma often need urgent incisional surgery, in which a glaucoma drainage device is implanted into the eye to improve aqueous outflow. Left untreated, neovascular glaucoma can quickly result in a blind painful eye, for which enucleation is indicated.

### What Else Can Look Like Diabetic Retinopathy?

Other retinal vascular diseases such as radiation retinopathy, sickle cell retinopathy (SCR), and hypertensive retinopathy can mimic diabetic retinopathy.

Exposure to ionizing radiation, either external beam or local plaque therapy, can damage the retina and cause microangiographic abnormalities similar to diabetic retinopathy. Fundus examination of radiation retinopathy shows cotton-wool spots, microaneurysms, retinal hemorrhages, macular edema, and neovascularization that are indistinguishable from diabetic retinopathy.[32] In suspected cases, it is important to elicit a history of radiation to differentiate the diagnoses.

SCR is caused by arteriolar and capillary occlusion. Like diabetic retinopathy, SCR is also classified as nonproliferative versus proliferative. Although sickle cell disease results in more systemic complications, proliferative SCR is more commonly associated with sickle cell hemoglobin C (Hb SC) and sickle cell thalassemia (SThal). Patients with SCR may lose vision because of macular ischemia, vitreous hemorrhage, and tractional retinal detachment.[33]

Hypertensive retinopathy can also feature similar retinal microvascular signs, which are predictive of incident stroke, congestive heart failure, and cardiovascular mortality.[34] Patients may present with acute bilateral blurry vision during a hypertensive crisis. Vision loss in this setting usually recovers with blood pressure control.

## How Else Does Diabetes Affect the Eye?

Diabetes can affect other structures of the eye apart from the retina, such as the cornea, the crystalline lens, and the cranial nerves. Thus, it is important for patients with diabetes to have a comprehensive eye evaluation in addition to the dilated fundus examination.

Diabetic neuropathy can affect cranial nerve V, causing corneal hypoesthesia or anesthesia, leading to neurotrophic keratopathy. This can present as persistent or recurrent corneal epithelial defects which may in turn increase the risk of corneal infection and perforation.[35] Patients with diabetes are at risk of poor healing after any ophthalmic surgery that involves the cornea such as cataract surgery or LASIK.[36]

Buildup of glucose in the aqueous humor and the crystalline lens can impair the lens' clarity, refractive index, and accommodative amplitude.[37] Patients with poorly controlled diabetes may therefore present with fluctuating blurry vision because of acute myopic shifts. Over time, prolonged hyperglycemia in the aqueous humor will also predispose patients to cataract formation. Patients with both type 1 and type 2 diabetes have a higher prevalence of cataracts than the general population. Patients with poorly controlled type 1 diabetes are at risk of subacute loss of vision in both eyes due to what are called bilateral snowflake cataracts. Patients with type 2 diabetes, on the other hand, develop typical age-related cataracts at a slightly earlier onset.[38]

Microvascular ischemia caused by diabetes can also manifest as cranial nerve vasculopathy, mostly commonly affecting cranial nerve VI. Patients present with double vision because of inability to abduct the affected eye. Diabetic ischemic cranial nerve palsies typically resolve within 4 to 6 months.[39]

Ischemia of cranial nerve II may present acutely as diabetic papillopathy, which may progress to optic atrophy in the late phase. Patients present with a pale optic nerve head, a relative afferent pupil defect, decreased vision, loss of color vision, and visual field loss. Unfortunately, there is no treatment for diabetic papillopathy or optic atrophy.[40]

## OTHER RETINAL VASCULAR DISEASES

In addition to diabetic retinopathy, there are many other retinal vascular diseases that are associated with systemic conditions. This section discusses two entities that are commonly encountered in eye clinic: retinal vein occlusion (RVO) and retinal artery occlusion (RAO).

## Retinal Vein Occlusion

RVO is the second leading cause of blindness from retinal vascular disease after diabetic retinopathy, and affects more than 16 million people worldwide.[41] RVO is further classified as central retinal vein occlusion (CRVO) or branch retinal vein occlusion (BRVO) based on the location of the obstruction.

### What causes central or branch retinal vein occlusion?

Both CRVO and BRVO are acute events caused by thrombus formation. In CRVO, a thrombus obstructs the central retinal vein, leading to vascular congestion, intraretinal hemorrhages, capillary nonperfusion, and capillary leakage. In BRVO, a branch retinal artery—thickened by arteriosclerosis—mechanically compresses a branch retinal vein at an arteriovenous crossing, leading to venous stasis and subsequent thrombus formation. The same downstream cascade of events resulting from vascular congestion then ensues, but the damage is isolated to the part of the retina being drained by the branch retinal vein.[42]

*Who gets central or branch retinal vein occlusion?*
CRVO and BRVO classically present in elderly patients with vascular risk factors. The cumulative prevalence of RVOs of both types is about 0.5% in patients older than age 40. The Eye Disease Case-Control Study Group (EDDC) identified risks factors for CRVO and BRVO.[43,44] Systemic risk factors for CRVO include hypertension, diabetes, smoking, and age. Systemic risk factors for BRVO include hypertension, cardiovascular disease, increased body mass index before age 20, and hypercoagulopathy/hyperviscosity.

For patients older than age 50 presenting with RVO who have known vascular risk factors, further workup to rule out underlying systemic precipitants of the RVO is not necessary. For younger, healthy patients, and particularly those presenting with bilateral RVOs, an underlying hypercoagulopathy/hyperviscosity syndrome or systemic vasculitis should be ruled out. Potential etiologies for RVO caused by an underlying systemic disease include:

- Hyperviscosity syndromes, such as leukemia, polycythemia vera, Waldenstrom macroglobinemia, and multiple myeloma
- Hypercoagulopathy, including factor V Leiden mutation, protein C deficiency, protein S deficiency, anticardiolipin antibody, antiphospholipid antibody, homocystinuria, and prothrombin mutation
- Vasculitis, including lupus, sarcoid, syphilis, and Behcet's disease

*How does central and branch retinal vein occlusion cause vision loss?*
Patients with RVO often present with acute painless vision loss and require urgent evaluation to establish the diagnosis. The severity of vision loss depends on the degree of retinal ischemia and presence or absence of macular edema. In CRVO, dilated fundus examination typically shows diffuse intraretinal hemorrhages, cotton-wool spots, and diffuse engorged and tortuous veins (**Fig. 9**). Macular edema is often present.[45] Similar findings are seen in BRVO, although limited to one area of the retina (**Fig. 10**), and macular edema is present only in about half of these patients.[46]

Over time, retinal ischemia can lead to the development of neovascularization of the optic nerve head, retina, angle, and iris. Retinal ischemia is more severe in patients

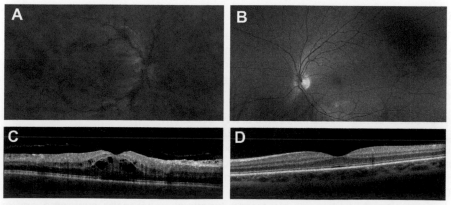

**Fig. 9.** CRVO. (*A*) Fundus photograph of the right eye shows diffuse intraretinal hemorrhages consistent an acute CRVO. (*B*) Fundus photograph of the unaffected left eye. (*C*) Optical coherence tomography (OCT) image shows macular edema, which may present in the acute phase of CRVO. (*D*) OCT image of the unaffected left eye with normal retina.

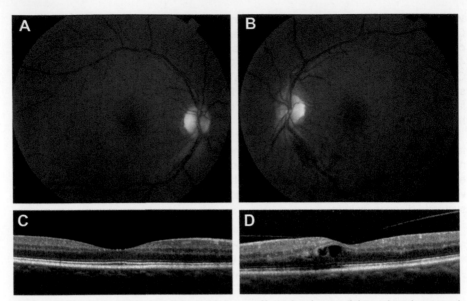

**Fig. 10.** BRVO. (*A*) Fundus photograph of the unaffected right eye. (*B*) Fundus photograph of the left eye with intraretinal hemorrhages in the inferior retina consistent with an inferior BRVO. (*C*) OCT image of the unaffected right eye with normal retina. (*D*) OCT image of the left eye with macula edema caused by BRVO.

with CRVO, who are more likely to develop complications from neovascularization. The presence of neovascularization is an indication for treatment with laser photocoagulation, as there are many potential vision-threatening complications from neovascularization (e.g., vitreous hemorrhage, retinal detachment, and neovascular glaucoma). In addition to neovascularization, both CRVO and BRVO may leave patients with chronic risk of recurrent macular edema requiring long-term management. The treatment for RVO-related macular edema is similar to treatment of diabetic macular edema, with anti-VEGF agents being first-line, followed by intravitreal corticosteroids and/or laser photocoagulation.[47,48]

## Retinal Artery Occlusion

Retinal artery occlusion is a medical emergency wherein the central retinal artery delivering blood supply to the inner layers of the retina or any of its branch tributaries is obstructed.[49] Similar to retinal vein occlusion, the severity of retinal arterial occlusive disease depends on the vessel involved (i.e., whether the occlusion is of the central retinal artery or a branch retinal artery).

### What causes central or branch retinal artery occlusion?

Both central retinal artery occlusion (CRAO) and branch retinal artery occlusion (BRAO) are caused by embolic and/or thrombotic occlusion. Retinal artery occlusion in patients of any age is often a sign of serious underlying systemic disease and should prompt a thorough evaluation. Older patients require evaluation for giant cell arteritis (GCA), as well as stroke workup including carotid ultrasound, echocardiogram, and brain imaging. A workup for hypercoagulopathy/hyperviscosity syndrome and/or vasculitis is recommended for afflicted younger patients.

Common causes of emboli associated with cardiovascular diseases include cholesterol emboli (i.e., Hollenhorst plaque) originating from the carotid arteries, platelet-fibrin emboli originating from atherosclerotic plaques, and calcific emboli originating from cardiac valves.

Other thromboembolic etiologies include:

- Fat emboli from long-bone fractures
- Septic emboli from infectious endocarditis
- Talc emboli from intravenous drug use
- Cardiac myxoma
- Arrhythmias
- Mitral valve prolapse
- Oral contraceptive use or pregnancy
- Coagulation disorders
- Sickle cell disease
- Retinal vasculitis
- Connective tissue disorders

### How does central or branch retinal artery occlusion cause vision loss?

In CRAO, obstruction of the central retinal artery impairs blood flow to most of the retina, and patients present with sudden, severe, painless loss of vision. The ischemic retina becomes edematous and appears opaque. The orange-red color of the choroidal vasculature beneath the foveola produces the appearance of the classic cherry-red spot in the center of the opaque macula. In the acute phase, OCT imaging shows diffuse hyper-reflectivity and loss of internal layer definition (**Fig. 11**). The central retinal artery eventually recanalizes with resolution of retinal edema, but the vision loss persists as the retina becomes atrophic. Most patients have permanent vision deficits worse than 20/400.[50,51] If there is a patent cilioretinal artery, present in about 20% of the general population, the patient may have some degree of central vision.

In BRAO, the obstruction occurs at one of the branch retinal arteries, leading to edema and opacification of the inner retina in the distribution of the affected vessel (**Fig. 12**). Patients with BRAO present with a visual field defect, which will also remain permanent even once the occluded vessel recanalizes and the edema resolves. Because of retinal ischemia, patients with CRAO and BRAO are also at risk of neovascularization, although less so compared to those with retinal vein occlusions.[52,53] The presence of neovascularization should prompt consideration for combined artery and vein occlusion, ophthalmic artery occlusion, or ocular ischemic syndrome.

### How are central and branch retinal artery occlusion managed?

Acute painless vision loss concerning for retinal artery occlusion requires immediate admission to an emergency department because of the high risk of ischemic stroke.[54] In particular, an elderly patient presenting with a CRAO needs emergent evaluation for GCA, which accounts for 1% to 2% of CRAO cases.[55] At minimum, serum erythrocyte sedimentation rate (ESR), C-reactive protein (CRP), and a complete blood count should be obtained. An elevated platelet count in the setting of elevated ESR and CRP is suggestive of GCA. In patients with suspected GCA, prompt initiation of high-dose systemic corticosteroids is recommended to prevent vision loss in the other eye.

Unfortunately, there are no proven treatments for vision loss caused by retinal artery occlusion. Potential treatments including ocular massage, anterior chamber paracentesis, hyperbaric oxygen therapy, and catheterization of the ophthalmic artery with tissue plasminogen activator have not been successful. Patients are monitored closely and treated with laser photocoagulation if they develop retinal or iris neovascularization.[49]

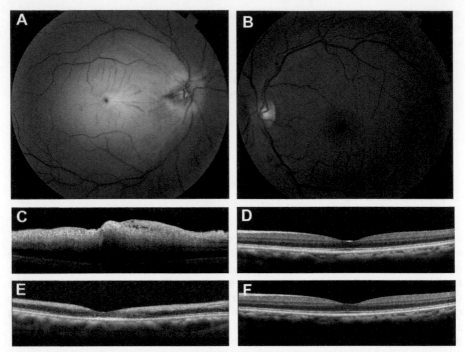

**Fig. 11.** CRAO. (*A*) Fundus photograph of the right eye shows diffuse retinal whitening and a cherry-red spot consistent with an acute CRAO. (*B*) Fundus photograph of the unaffected left eye. (*C*) OCT image of the right eye shows edema and opacification of the inner retinal layers during the acute phase of CRAO. (*E*) OCT image of the right eye shows thinning of the retina 6 weeks later in the late phase of the CRAO. (*D, F*) OCT images of the unaffected left eye with normal retina.

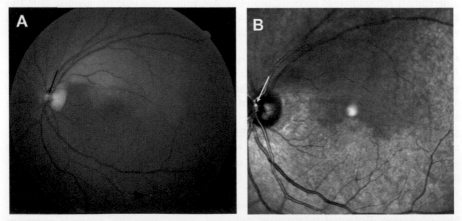

**Fig. 12.** BRAO. (*A*) Fundus photograph of the left eye shows segmental opacification of the retina consistent with a superior BRAO. In addition to the causative embolus seen near the branching point (*black arrow*), there is also a smaller embolus in the distal inferior vascular arcade (*arrowhead*). (*B*) Near-infrared reflectance imaging highlights the causative embolus near the branching point at the optic nerve head (*yellow arrow*).

## SUMMARY

The retinal vasculature is most commonly afflicted by uncontrolled diabetes but is also susceptible to thromboembolic insults associated with other systemic diseases. Both the internists and medical subspecialists play a crucial role in the prevention, detection, evaluation, and management of vision-threatening retinal vascular diseases.

## CLINICS CARE POINTS

- Intensive glycemic control can prevent vision loss from diabetic retinopathy.
- Patients with diabetes who are pregnant require more frequent eye examinations.
- Regular dilated eye examinations by an ophthalmologist or via telemedicine screening offered by primary care physicians and/or medical subspecialists can provide convenient and timely diabetic retinopathy screening.
- For patients with diabetic retinopathy with poor access to follow-up care, early treatment with laser photocoagulation could be sight-saving.
- Systemic anticoagulants may be continued in patients with intraocular bleeding from diabetic retinopathy.
- Diabetic retinopathy can be mimicked by retinopathy caused by hypertension, radiation, and sickle cell disease.
- Patients with diabetes should be counseled that in addition to diabetic retinopathy, poorly controlled disease can also cause vision loss due to corneal ulceration, cataracts, cranial nerve palsy, and ischemic optic neuropathy.
- Retinal vein occlusion in young patients and in those without known vascular risk factors warrant a systemic work-up to identify potential underlying precipitants.
- Acute painless vision loss concerning for retinal artery occlusion requires immediate admission to an emergency department because of the high risk of ischemic stroke.
- Elderly patients presenting with retinal artery occlusion should be evaluated for GCA in addition to emergent stroke workup.

## DISCLOSURE

The authors have nothing to disclose.

## REFERENCES

1. Klein BE. Overview of epidemiologic studies of diabetic retinopathy. Ophthalmic Epidemiol 2007;14(4):179–83.
2. Saeedi P, Petersohn I, Salpea P, et al. Global and regional diabetes prevalence estimates for 2019 and projections for 2030 and 2045: Results from the International Diabetes Federation Diabetes Atlas, 9(th) edition. Diabetes Res Clin Pract 2019;157:107843.
3. Yau JW, Rogers SL, Kawasaki R, et al. Global prevalence and major risk factors of diabetic retinopathy. Diabetes Care 2012;35(3):556–64.
4. International Diabetes Federation. Diabetes: facts and figures. Available at: https://www.idf.org/our-activities/care-prevention/eye-health.html.     Accessed August 23, 2020.
5. Centers for Disease Control and Prevention. National diabetes statistics Report, 2020. Atlanta, GA: Centers for Disease Control and Prevention, US Dept of Health

and Human Services; 2020. Available at: https://www.cdc.gov/diabetes/pdfs/data/statistics/national-diabetes-statistics-report.pdf.

6. National Eye Institute. Diabetic Retinopathy Data and Statistics. Available at: https://www.nei.nih.gov/learn-about-eye-health/resources-for-health-educators/eye-health-data-and-statistics/diabetic-retinopathy-data-and-statistics. Accessed August 23, 2020.

7. Klein R, Lee KE, Knudtson MD, et al. Changes in visual impairment prevalence by period of diagnosis of diabetes: the Wisconsin Epidemiologic Study of Diabetic Retinopathy. Ophthalmology 2009;116(10):1937–42.

8. The relationship of glycemic exposure (HbA1c) to the risk of development and progression of retinopathy in the diabetes control and complications trial. Diabetes 1995;44(8):968–83.

9. Tight blood pressure control and risk of macrovascular and microvascular complications in type 2 diabetes: UKPDS 38. UK Prospective Diabetes Study Group. BMJ 1998;317(7160):703–13.

10. Antonetti DA, Klein R, Gardner TW. Diabetic retinopathy. N Engl J Med 2012; 366(13):1227–39.

11. American Academy of Ophthalmology Retina/Vitreous Panel. Preferred Practice Pattern Guidelines. Diabetic retinopathy. San Francisco: American Academy of Ophthalmology; 2019. Available at: https://www.aao.org/preferred-practice-pattern/diabetic-retinopathy-ppp.

12. Wang SY, Andrews CA, Herman WH, et al. Incidence and risk factors for developing diabetic retinopathy among youths with type 1 or type 2 diabetes throughout the United States. Ophthalmology 2017;124(4):424–30.

13. Early photocoagulation for diabetic retinopathy. ETDRS report number 9. Early Treatment Diabetic Retinopathy Study Research Group. Ophthalmology 1991; 98(5 Suppl):766–85.

14. Group AS, Group AES, Chew EY, et al. Effects of medical therapies on retinopathy progression in type 2 diabetes. N Engl J Med 2010;363(3):233–44.

15. The effect of intensive diabetes therapy on the development and progression of neuropathy. The Diabetes Control and Complications Trial Research Group. Ann Intern Med 1995;122(8):561–8.

16. Diabetic Retinopathy Study Research Group. Preliminary report on effects of photocoagulation therapy. Am J Ophthalmol 2018;185:14–24.

17. Gross JG, Glassman AR, Liu D, et al. Five-year outcomes of panretinal photocoagulation vs intravitreous ranibizumab for proliferative diabetic retinopathy: a randomized clinical trial. JAMA Ophthalmol 2018;136(10):1138–48.

18. Centers for Disease Control and Prevention. Diabetes Report card 2017. Atlanta (GA): Centers for Disease Control and Prevention, US Dept of Health and Human Services; 2020. Available at: https://www.cdc.gov/diabetes/pdfs/library/diabetesreportcard2017-508.pdf.

19. Photocoagulation for diabetic macular edema: Early Treatment Diabetic Retinopathy Study report no. 4. The Early Treatment Diabetic Retinopathy Study Research Group. Int Ophthalmol Clin 1987;27(4):265–72.

20. Owsley C, McGwin G Jr, Lee DJ, et al. Diabetes eye screening in urban settings serving minority populations: detection of diabetic retinopathy and other ocular findings using telemedicine. JAMA Ophthalmol 2015;133(2):174–81.

21. Mansberger SL, Sheppler C, Barker G, et al. Long-term comparative effectiveness of telemedicine in providing diabetic retinopathy screening examinations: a randomized clinical trial. JAMA Ophthalmol 2015;133(5):518–25.

22. Jani PD, Forbes L, Choudhury A, et al. Evaluation of diabetic retinal screening and factors for ophthalmology referral in a telemedicine network. JAMA Ophthalmol 2017;135(7):706–14.
23. Gibson DM. Estimates of the percentage of US adults with diabetes who could be screened for diabetic retinopathy in primary care settings. JAMA Ophthalmol 2019;137(4):440–4.
24. Varma R, Bressler NM, Doan QV, et al. Prevalence of and risk factors for diabetic macular edema in the United States. JAMA Ophthalmol 2014;132(11):1334–40.
25. Wells JA, Glassman AR, Ayala AR, et al. Aflibercept, bevacizumab, or ranibizumab for diabetic macular edema: two-year results from a comparative effectiveness randomized clinical trial. Ophthalmology 2016;123(6):1351–9.
26. Ryan EH Jr, Han DP, Ramsay RC, et al. Diabetic macular edema associated with glitazone use. Retina 2006;26(5):562–70.
27. Samara WA, Shahlaee A, Adam MK, et al. Quantification of diabetic macular ischemia using optical coherence tomography angiography and its relationship with visual acuity. Ophthalmology 2017;124(2):235–44.
28. Chew EY, Klein ML, Murphy RP, et al. Effects of aspirin on vitreous/preretinal hemorrhage in patients with diabetes mellitus. Early Treatment Diabetic Retinopathy Study report no. 20. Arch Ophthalmol 1995;113(1):52–5.
29. Early vitrectomy for severe vitreous hemorrhage in diabetic retinopathy. Four-year results of a randomized trial: Diabetic Retinopathy Vitrectomy Study Report 5. Arch Ophthalmol 1990;108(7):958–64.
30. Brunner S, Binder S. Surgery for proliferative diabetic retinopathy. In: Schachat AP, Wilkinson CP, Hinton DR, et al, editors. Ryan's retina, vol. 3, 6th edition. Philadelphia: Elsevier/Saunders; 2018. Chapter 115. p. 2107-23.
31. Yang YF, Herbert L, Ruschen H, et al. Nitrous oxide anaesthesia in the presence of intraocular gas can cause irreversible blindness. BMJ 2002;325(7363):532–3.
32. Patel SJ, Schachat AP. Radiation retinopathy. In: Albert DM, Miller JW, Azar DT, et al, editors. Albert & Jakobiec's principles and practice of ophthalmology. 3rd edition. Philadelphia: Saunders; 2008. Chapter 175. p. 2207-10.
33. Elagouz M, Jyothi S, Gupta B, et al. Sickle cell disease and the eye: old and new concepts. Surv Ophthalmol 2010;55(4):359–77.
34. Wong TY, Mitchell P. The eye in hypertension. Lancet 2007;369(9559):425–35.
35. Lockwood A, Hope-Ross M, Chell P. Neurotrophic keratopathy and diabetes mellitus. Eye (Lond) 2006;20(7):837–9.
36. Simpson RG, Moshirfar M, Edmonds JN, et al. Laser in-situ keratomileusis in patients with diabetes mellitus: a review of the literature. Clin Ophthalmol 2012;6:1665–74.
37. Hejtmancik JF, Riazuddin SA, McGreal R, et al. Lens Biology and Biochemistry. Prog Mol Biol Transl Sci 2015;134:169–201.
38. Flynn HW Jr, Smiddy WE, editors. Diabetes and ocular disease: past, present, and future therapies. Ophthalmology monograph 14. San Francisco: American Academy of Ophthalmology;; 2000.
39. Tamhankar MA, Biousse V, Ying GS, et al. Isolated third, fourth, and sixth cranial nerve palsies from presumed microvascular versus other causes: a prospective study. Ophthalmology 2013;120(11):2264–9.
40. Bayraktar Z, Alacali N, Bayraktar S. Diabetic papillopathy in type II diabetic patients. Retina 2002;22(6):752–8.
41. Rogers S, McIntosh RL, Cheung N, et al. The prevalence of retinal vein occlusion: pooled data from population studies from the United States, Europe, Asia, and Australia. Ophthalmology 2010;117(2):313–319 e1.

42. Ho M, Liu DT, Lam DS, et al. Retinal Vein Occlusions, from Basics to the Latest Treatment. Retina 2016;36(3):432–48.
43. Risk factors for branch retinal vein occlusion. The Eye Disease Case-control Study Group. Am J Ophthalmol 1993;116(3):286–96.
44. Risk factors for central retinal vein occlusion. The Eye Disease Case-Control Study Group. Arch Ophthalmol 1996;114(5):545–54.
45. Natural history and clinical management of central retinal vein occlusion. The Central Vein Occlusion Study Group. Arch Ophthalmol 1997;115(4):486–91.
46. Argon laser photocoagulation for macular edema in branch vein occlusion. The Branch Vein Occlusion Study Group. Am J Ophthalmol 1984;98(3):271–82.
47. Ehlers JP, Kim SJ, Yeh S, et al. Therapies for macular edema associated with branch retinal vein occlusion: a report by the American Academy of Ophthalmology. Ophthalmology 2017;124(9):1412–23.
48. Yeh S, Kim SJ, Ho AC, et al. Therapies for macular edema associated with central retinal vein occlusion: a report by the American Academy of Ophthalmology. Ophthalmology 2015;122(4):769–78.
49. American Academy of Ophthalmology Retina/Vitreous Panel. Preferred Practice® Pattern Guidelines. Retinal and ophthalmic artery occlusion. San Francisco: American Academy of Ophthalmology; 2019. Available at: https://www.aao.org/preferred-practice-pattern/retinal-ophthalmic-artery-occlusions-ppp.
50. Ahn SJ, Woo SJ, Park KH, et al. Retinal and choroidal changes and visual outcome in central retinal artery occlusion: an optical coherence tomography study. Am J Ophthalmol 2015;159(4):667–76.
51. Hayreh SS, Zimmerman MB. Central retinal artery occlusion: visual outcome. Am J Ophthalmol 2005;140(3):376–91.
52. Jung YH, Ahn SJ, Hong JH, et al. Incidence and clinical features of neovascularization of the iris following acute central retinal artery occlusion. Korean J Ophthalmol 2016;30(5):352–9.
53. Duker JS, Brown GC. The efficacy of panretinal photocoagulation for neovascularization of the iris after central retinal artery obstruction. Ophthalmology 1989;96(1):92–5.
54. Kernan WN, Ovbiagele B, Black HR, et al. Guidelines for the prevention of stroke in patients with stroke and transient ischemic attack: a guideline for healthcare professionals from the American Heart Association/American Stroke Association. Stroke 2014;45(7):2160–236.
55. Hayreh SS. Ocular vascular occlusive disorders: natural history of visual outcome. Prog Retin Eye Res 2014;41:1–25.

# Age-Related Macular Degeneration

Catherine J. Thomas, MD, MHA, MS, Rukhsana G. Mirza, MD, MS,
Manjot K. Gill, MD, FRCS (C)*

## KEYWORDS

- Drusen • Choroidal neovascularization (CNV)
- Vascular endothelial growth factor (VEGF)
- Neovascular (exudative, wet) age-related macular degeneration
- Nonneovascular (nonexudative, dry) age-related macular degeneration
- Geographic atrophy

## KEY POINTS

- Age-related macular degeneration is a leading cause of irreversible vision loss globally.
- Dilated fundus examination should be performed on individuals over the age of 55 to screen for age-related macular degeneration.
- Age, smoking history, hyperlipidemia, family history, and ethnicity are all risk factors for developing age-related macular degeneration.
- Ophthalmologists generally do not advise cessation of systemic antiplatelet/anticoagulation therapies, but discussion with the prescribing physician may be warranted in certain clinical scenarios.
- There is no cure for age-related macular degeneration; however, intravitreal injections are the gold-standard treatment for advanced neovascular disease.

## INTRODUCTION

Age-related macular degeneration (AMD) affects millions of people worldwide and is a leading cause of blindness globally.[1] There are 2 main types of AMD, neovascular and nonneovascular AMD, which can be further classified based on specific features of the disease. Nonneovascular AMD ("dry" AMD) accounts for almost 80% to 85% of all cases and generally carries a more favorable visual prognosis. Neovascular AMD ("wet" AMD) affects the remaining 15% to 20% and accounts for approximately 80% of severe vision loss as a result of AMD.[2]

Department of Ophthalmology, Feinberg School of Medicine, Northwestern University, 645 North Michigan Avenue, Suite 440, Chicago, IL 60611, USA
* Corresponding author.
*E-mail address:* mgill@nm.org
Twitter: @CJThomasMD (C.J.T.); @rg-mirza (R.G.M.); @ManjotGillMD (M.K.G.)

Med Clin N Am 105 (2021) 473–491
https://doi.org/10.1016/j.mcna.2021.01.003     **medical.theclinics.com**
0025-7125/21/© 2021 The Authors. Published by Elsevier Inc. This is an open access article under the CC BY-NC-ND license (http://creativecommons.org/licenses/by-nc-nd/4.0/).

## BACKGROUND

AMD involves pathologic changes to the deeper retinal layers of the macula and surrounding vasculature resulting in central vision loss. The accumulation of retinal deposits, called drusen, are a hallmark clinical finding in AMD (described in later discussion) and may be the first sign of the "dry" form of the disease. Dry AMD is the most common morphologic type and may progress to "wet" or neovascular AMD, whereby central choroidal neovascular membranes (CNV) can lead to hemorrhaging and exudation in the retina and profound vision loss. These membranes form as a result of abnormal vascular proliferation or angiogenesis owing to the release of vascular endothelial growth factor (VEGF). The treatment of choice for these lesions is intravitreal injections with anti–vascular endothelial growth factor (anti-VEGF) therapy, which has revolutionized the management of advanced AMD. Another variant of late AMD is the "dry" or nonexudative type, whereby geographic atrophy or atrophic scars develop in the macula. These atrophic lesions do not respond to anti-VEGF therapy and have similarly devastating permanent effects on visual function if involving the fovea.

AMD is the leading cause of irreversible blindness in the developed world in individuals over the age of 60.[3] Consequences of poor vision include increased risk of fall, depression, and the need for long-term care if unable to perform activities of daily living, such as dressing, eating, and working.[4] The direct cost of AMD to the North American health care system was more than 250 billion dollars in 2008 with a steady increase in the number of new cases annually.[5] The aging population indicates that these numbers will continue to increase at an exponential rate. The visual implications of AMD can exacerbate the already challenging health-related concerns and comorbidities of the elderly and significantly impact quality of life. Understanding the basic signs and symptoms of AMD is useful in counseling patients on when to seek ophthalmologic care and prevent further vision loss.

Although there is no cure for AMD, preventative and proactive measures are crucial. Disease progression can be slowed by addressing certain modifiable risk factors, such as smoking, diet, and cardiovascular disease.[6] The Age-Related Eye Disease Study (AREDS) led to the development of a specific combination of vitamin supplementation for the prevention of disease progression for patients with specific characteristics of AMD.[7] There are several subtypes of AMD, not all of which respond to anti-VEGF therapy or meet criteria for recommending AREDS vitamins. The prognosis is variable depending on the stage of the disease. Timely referral for ophthalmologic care is important for the treatment and prevention of the long-term sequelae of AMD.

## EPIDEMIOLOGY

Almost 200 million people worldwide have some form of AMD.[3] In the United States, the numbers exceed 10 million and are steadily increasing.[5] Age is the main risk factor for developing AMD; however, cigarette smoking, increased body mass index, hypertension, hyperlipidemia, and genetics are other important risk factors.[8,9] The US Twin Study of Age-Related Macular Degeneration examined cigarette smoking and omega-3 fatty acid intake in elderly male twins and demonstrated that both current smokers and those with a past history of smoking had an almost 2-fold increased risk of developing AMD.[10] Other studies suggest a 4-fold increase in the risk of developing AMD for smokers.[11] The Rotterdam Study demonstrated that former smokers are at an increased risk even after 20 years of abstinence from cigarettes.[12] Conversely, dietary omega-3 fatty acids and omega-6 fatty acids most commonly found in fish were found to be protective against AMD.[10] Several studies have shown an increased risk of AMD in individuals with hypertension possibly because of the impact of systolic blood pressure on choroidal blood flow.[13] Hyperlipidemia as a risk factor for AMD has also been widely examined with some investigators, suggesting that elevated high-density lipoprotein and high cholesterol intake may be associated with neovascular AMD and elevated serum cholesterol with the development of geographic atrophy.[13] Studies on gender predilection have been inconclusive, although a female preponderance for AMD has been reported in the literature.[14]

Wong and colleagues[3] reported the prevalence of AMD across ethnicities. Findings showed that those of European ancestry were more likely to develop early, intermediate, and advanced AMD compared with Asians and Africans. Europeans were also more likely to develop geographic atrophy than Asians, Hispanics, and Africans.[3] Although Hispanics are considered lower risk for AMD compared with whites, the Los Angeles Latino Eye Study found the prevalence of AMD to be greater than 8% in Latinos over 80 years old.[15]

## SIGNS AND SYMPTOMS

There may be minimal to no symptoms associated with early and intermediate AMD whereby there are predominantly small- and medium-sized drusen deposited in the macula. Patients may note subtle changes, such as distortion (metamorphopsia), increased blurring at near, particularly while reading, and decreased contrast sensitivity. The presence of neovascular AMD generally leads to more rapid and profound visual symptoms that may be acute or gradually worsen. These symptoms include severe distortion and/or a large central scotoma or blind spot owing to retinal hemorrhage and fluid accumulation. Patients may complain of difficulty recognizing faces. Patients with geographic atrophy may also note similar symptoms of distortion and central scotoma. The Amsler grid[16] was developed as a self-monitoring tool for patients to test each eye independently, looking for distortion or the presence of a scotoma that may indicate progression from dry to wet or neovascular AMD.

## OVERVIEW AND CLASSIFICATION

AMD is defined by the presence of specific changes in the macula particularly the deposition of focal yellow extracellular deposits known as drusen. The presence of macular drusen may be the first sign of the dry form of the disease, and patients may often be asymptomatic (**Fig. 1**). The size and number of drusen contribute to the risk of disease progression. Small drusen are classified as less than 63 μm in diameter, medium drusen 63 to 124 μm, and large drusen ≥125 μm.[17] Drusen may also be described as hard or soft, whereby hard drusen have discrete borders and are often small. Soft drusen have less distinct borders and may become confluent to form larger, more high-risk lesions.[17] The Beaver Dam Eye Study demonstrated an incidence close to 30% for the development of advanced AMD in patients with the presence of larger soft drusen.[18,19] The classification of AMD is divided into early, intermediate, and advanced nonneovascular AMD or advanced neovascular AMD (**Table 1**). The presence of small macular drusen or few medium-sized drusen poses a lower risk in terms of progression to advanced AMD and may not lead to vision loss. Pigmentary changes in the macula may also be a sign of early disease and serve as a predictor of progression to more advanced AMD.[18] Many medium-sized drusen or 1 large drusen, defined as intermediate AMD, confers a higher risk for progression to advanced disease with more judicious monitoring recommended (**Fig. 2**).

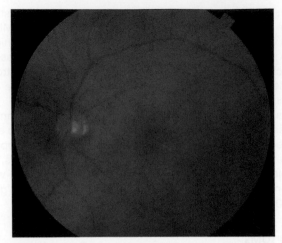

**Fig. 1.** Macular drusen of the left eye. (Image courtesy of R. Mirza, M.D.)

## Wet Versus Dry Age-Related Macular Degeneration

There are certain morphologic features to further categorize AMD based on the presence or absence of abnormal CNV proliferation or the presence or absence of atrophic lesions referred to as geographic atrophy. "Dry" (nonexudative or nonneovascular) AMD refers to both the presence of drusen in either early or intermediate disease and also the atrophic variant of dry AMD whereby geographic atrophy is the predominant feature (**Fig. 3**). The presence of geographic atrophy in the macula is categorized as advanced dry AMD when it involves the fovea and may lead to progressive permanent vision loss, as these lesions often advance over time. Atrophic changes occur because of loss of outer retinal tissue and the surrounding vascular network, specifically the retinal pigment epithelial (RPE) layer, Bruch membrane, and the choriocapillaris. Advanced dry AMD is thought to be due in part to inflammatory and degenerative insults that lead to subsequent photoreceptor loss.[20]

"Wet" (exudative or neovascular) AMD is the most common form of advanced AMD.[18] The neovascularization that develops leads to hemorrhaging and leakage of fluid in the inner retinal layers or subretinal space, ultimately causing fibrosis and permanent vision loss in the absence of treatment (**Figs. 4** and **5**). The early or intermediate forms of dry AMD may have a more favorable prognosis if the disease course

**Table 1**
Classification of age-related macular degeneration based on the Age-Related Eye Disease Study[19]

| Early AMD | Intermediate AMD | Advanced Nonneovascular AMD (Advanced Dry AMD) | Advanced Neovascular AMD (Wet AMD) |
|---|---|---|---|
| Presence of small drusen or few medium-sized drusen in 1 or both eyes Pigmentary changes | Presence of many medium-sized drusen, 1 large drusen, and/or geographic atrophy not involving the central macula (fovea) | Geographic atrophy involving the central macula or fovea | Choroidal neovascularization in 1 eye |

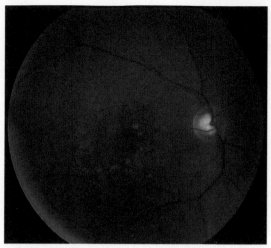

**Fig. 2.** Intermediate AMD. (Image courtesy of R. Mirza, M.D.)

remains stable. It is important to be aware that for all forms of dry AMD there is a 10% to 15% risk of progression to wet AMD[21] at some point throughout the disease course. There may also be overlap in both atrophic and neovascular features, where wet or neovascular AMD progresses to geographic atrophy and vice versa.[22] Many practitioners and patients are concerned about continuing systemic anticoagulation/antiplatelet medications in cases of neovascular AMD. An epidemiologic review demonstrated an increased risk of intraocular hemorrhage in those on systemic anticoagulants, specifically aspirin, clopidogrel, and warfarin; however, ophthalmologists do not advise cessation of these therapies, especially when used to treat life-threatening conditions.[23] A discussion may be warranted between the primary care

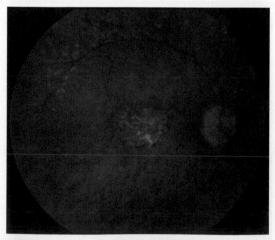

**Fig. 3.** Central geographic atrophy with drusen outside of the macula. (Image courtesy of R. Mirza, M.D.)

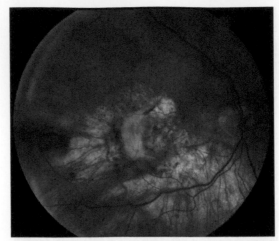

**Fig. 4.** Macular fibrosis and scar formation as a result of neovascular AMD. (Image courtesy of M. Gill, M.D.)

provider and the ophthalmologist in certain scenarios to evaluate the risks and benefit profile.

## PATHOPHYSIOLOGY

The retina is the transparent central nervous system tissue lining the inner aspect of the back wall of the eye and is essential for vision. There are multiple layers and components of the retina, each serving different functions. The central portion of the retina, termed the macula, refers to the multilayered area responsible for the most detailed aspects of human vision. The center of the macula, the fovea, is essential for maintaining basic visual function necessary to perform daily activities, such as facial recognition, reading, and driving (**Fig. 6**). AMD primarily affects the outer retina, which includes the RPE, Bruch membrane, the choriocapillaris, and underlying choroid

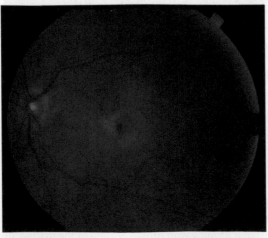

**Fig. 5.** Exudative AMD with hemorrhage and fluid accumulation involving the fovea. (Image courtesy of R. Mirza, M.D.)

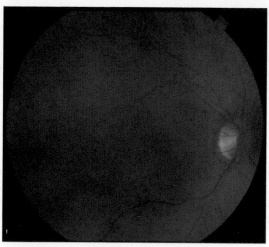

**Fig. 6.** Normal fundus photo of the right eye. (Image courtesy of M. Gill, M.D.)

(**Fig. 7**). The RPE maintains important homeostatic functions of the retina, including but not limited to nutrient absorption, phagocytosis, and electrolyte balance, whereas the choriocapillaris and choroid contain the rich vascular network that nourishes the outer layers of the retina.[24] Bruch membrane mediates interactions between the

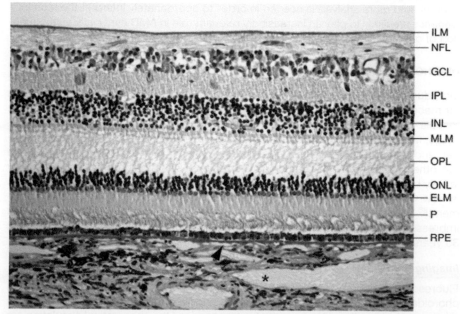

**Fig. 7.** Normal layers of the retina (periodic acid–Schiff [PAS] stain). ELM, external limiting membrane; GCL, ganglion cell layer; ILM, internal limiting membrane; INL, inner nuclear layer; IPL, inner plexiform layer; MLM, middle limiting membrane; NFL, nerve fiber layer; ONL, outer nuclear layer; OPL, outer plexiform layer; P, photoreceptors (inner/outer segments) of rods and cones. Bruch membrane, arrowhead; choroid, asterisk. © American Academy of Ophthalmology.

RPE and choriocapillaris and plays an important role in the development of neovascular lesions in AMD. The RPE nourishes the photoreceptor layer, where the rods and cones perform the intricate phototransduction process essential to visual function.[20] The dysfunction and atrophy of the RPE present in AMD impact the health of the photoreceptor layer and interferes with phototransduction. Such dysfunction leads to disruption of signal transmission from the retina to the brain and subsequent vision loss. In addition, the choroidal vasculature is thought to be affected by microvascular insults that occur in certain systemic diseases, such as hypertension and hyperlipidemia.[13] These microvascular insults suggest both an ischemic and an inflammatory component influencing the pathophysiology of the disease.

Abnormal angiogenesis is mediated by VEGF and plays a critical role in the development of CNV in advanced neovascular AMD. The normal retinal circulation requires VEGF for healthy choroidal and retinal vasculature. The abnormal expression of specific VEGF subtypes is induced by hypoxia and leads to the proliferation of new blood vessels susceptible to leakage and bleeding characteristic of neovascular AMD.[25]

### Genetics

There are many genes linked to the development of AMD.[26] The complement factor H gene was the first identified gene for susceptibility to AMD, whereby disruption in complement-mediated regulatory function is thought to play a role in the formation of drusen.[21] The noncomplement mediated age-related maculopathy susceptibility 2 gene is also associated with the development of AMD. At this time, routine genetic testing is not currently recommended, as the results do not support altering current treatment guidelines for advanced AMD. In addition, there are few qualified testing centers, and more analysis is needed in order to appropriately interpret the results.[27] Genetics are likely to play an increasingly relevant role in AMD especially as the function of genetic testing and gene therapy evolves.

## DIAGNOSIS

Individuals over 55 years of age should have a dilated fundus examination to screen for macular degeneration.[8] In order to diagnose AMD, the examiner will evaluate the macula for deposits of drusen, pigmentary changes, geographic atrophy, hemorrhage, fluid, exudate, scar formation, and fibrosis. Attention is given to the size, number, and distribution of drusen. A complete eye examination is also performed to rule out other coexisting ocular pathologic conditions. The staging of the disease may largely be based on the examination; however, use of a variety of imaging techniques is now considered essential to correlate examination findings and guide management.[28] Technological advancements in ophthalmology continue to progress at an impressive pace with retinal imaging modalities evolving significantly in the past 30 years.

### Imaging Modalities

Fluorescein angiography (FA) has historically been the gold standard for assessing choroidal neovascularization in AMD. It is an invasive procedure whereby fluorescein dye is injected into the vein of a patient, and images of the chorioretinal circulation are taken over the course of several minutes that may detect the presence of leakage from different types of neovascular lesions.[28] Indocyanine green angiography (ICG) is a similar method that may be performed in certain scenarios. ICG involves the injection of indocyanine green, a dye that is useful in evaluating the choroidal circulation, whereby occult CNV lesions may be detected.

Optical coherence tomography (OCT) is a widely used, noninvasive tool that allows for an in-depth display of each of the retinal layers and has revolutionized the understanding and management of AMD.[28] OCT is comparable to ultrasound but uses light rather than sound waves[29] to provide a detailed cross-sectional image of the 10 retinal layers and underlying choroid, allowing for visualization of the specific layers impacted by AMD (**Fig. 8**). The images help to differentiate between wet and dry AMD and allow the physician to better characterize disease stage and CNV activity. OCT may show fluid within and beneath the retina that is found in wet macular degeneration and can be compared longitudinally to assess response to treatment and guide management (**Figs. 9–11**).

A more recent imaging modality includes optical coherence tomography angiography (OCT-A). OCT-A is a noninvasive advancement that allows for better visualization of the rich vascular network of the choroid. This technique aids in the understanding of the microvascular changes that occur in the presence of CNV lesions in neovascular AMD. OCT-A also serves as a tool that may allow for earlier detection of neovascularization with the goal of closer monitoring and earlier intervention when appropriate.[30] In many cases, OCT-A has replaced FA and ICG.

## MANAGEMENT
### Laser Therapy

Before 2000, thermal laser therapy was the mainstay of treatment of wet AMD. Argon-laser photocoagulation leads to regression of CNV with scar formation through the use of thermal energy to directly target neovascular lesions.[31] A limitation of focal laser is the occurrence of scotoma or permanent central vision loss in the treated area.

Around the year 2000, photodynamic therapy (PDT) became available. PDT involves the intravenous injection of a photosensitizing dye (verteporfin) that travels throughout the body and accumulates in CNV and upon treatment with longer wavelength infrared laser can induce closure of CNV lesions. PDT is still used today as an adjuvant in cases refractory to anti-VEGF alone.

### Intravitreal Injections and Anti–Vascular Endothelial Growth Factor Agents

The development of localized intravitreal treatment with anti-VEGF therapy has revolutionized the treatment of AMD in addition to other diseases, whereby angiogenic factors play a role, such as diabetic retinopathy, venous occlusive disease, and other causes of choroidal neovascularization. The injections can be done quickly and seamlessly in office and require little to no recovery time for the patient with minimal risks and few side effects. The technique allows for the safe and direct delivery of the

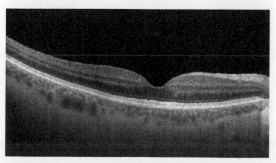

**Fig. 8.** Normal OCT of right eye showing intact retinal layers. (Image courtesy of M. Gill, M.D.)

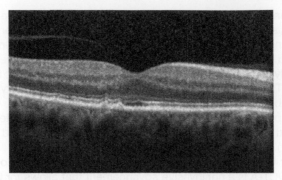

**Fig. 9.** Dry AMD with macular drusen. (Image courtesy of M. Gill, M.D.)

desired agent into the vitreous cavity using a small, 30-gauge needle through the pars plana, which lies 3 to 4 mm behind the limbus (**Fig. 12**). Topical anesthetic options are available for patient comfort, and povidone-iodine has proven to be safe and effective in the prevention of infection.[32] The volume of medication injected is generally 0.05 mL and is delivered in a prefilled syringe from the manufacturer or compounding pharmacy. Despite patients' perceptions and fears regarding intravitreal injections, most patients studied by Fallor and colleagues[33] thought that their vision was preserved and treatments were effective.

For wet AMD, anti-VEGF agents have proven to be beneficial in targeting CNV lesions and preserving vision.[34] VEGF is present throughout the body and required for normal angiogenesis. However, the pathologic upregulation of VEGF leads to leakage and neovascularization that develop in advanced AMD.[25] VEGF-A was one of the earliest mediators implicated in the development of CNV and an early target of anti-VEGF therapies. There are various isoforms of VEGF-A and additional angiogenic forms of VEGF, including VEGF-B and placental-like growth factor (PLGF). The 3 most widely used intravitreal agents for wet AMD include ranibizumab (Genentech), aflibercept (Regeneron), and bevacizumab (Genentech). Ranibizumab is a recombinant, humanized, monoclonal antibody fragment that neutralizes all forms of VEGF-A and was first approved for use in 2005. Aflibercept was Food and Drug Administration (FDA) approved in 2011 and is a VEGF-trap fusion protein that binds both VEGF-A and platelet-derived growth factor. Bevacizumab is a monoclonal

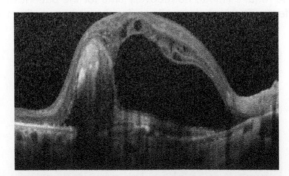

**Fig. 10.** OCT depicts neovascular AMD with significant intraretinal and subretinal fluid involving the macula and fovea with complete disruption of retinal architecture. (Image courtesy of M. Gill, M.D.)

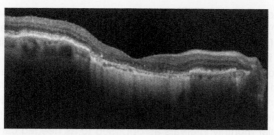

**Fig. 11.** Geographic atrophy at the center of the macula with loss of outer retinal layers. (Image courtesy of R. Mirza, M.D.)

antibody that binds to all VEGF-A isoforms and is used systemically in the treatment of colon cancer. Ranibizumab and aflibercept are both FDA approved for exudative AMD, while bevacizumab is used in an off-label manner and is a cost-effective alternative.

## Surgery

Surgical excision of neovascular lesions was previously described as an option but has largely been abandoned because of current minimally invasive, more successful treatments as described above. In the 1990s, the Submacular Surgery Trials investigated outcomes in patients with neovascular AMD who underwent submacular surgery for hemorrhage owing to CNV lesions. The outcomes of the study showed no benefit in the group that underwent surgery versus observation alone and demonstrated an increased rate of complications in the surgery arm.[35]

## Trials

There are several landmark clinical trials describing the efficacy of the 3 main anti-VEGF agents currently in use. MARINA (Minimally Classic/Occult Trial of the Anti-VEGF Antibody Ranibizumab in the Treatment of Neovascular AMD) and ANCHOR

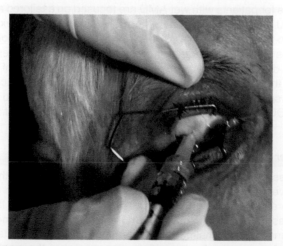

**Fig. 12.** Intravitreal injection technique. This image was originally published in the Retina Image Bank Web site. John T. Thompson, MD. Intravitreal injection of anti-VEGF Drug. Retina Image Bank. 2017; Image Number 27125. © the American Society of Retina Specialists.

(Anti-VEGF Antibody for the Treatment of Predominantly Classic Choroidal Neovascularization in AMD) evaluated the efficacy of monthly injections of ranibizumab. Both studies were the first to demonstrate a significant improvement in vision with regularly dosed injections in patients with exudative AMD.

The Comparison of AMD Treatment Trial (CATT) study compared the efficacy of ranibizumab and bevacizumab for the treatment of exudative AMD as well as compared differing treatment strategies. Both agents showed equivalent outcomes in terms of final visual acuity. The 2-year CATT study also demonstrated that receiving injections at regular monthly intervals as opposed to as needed can result in slightly better visual outcomes.[36] The efficacy of aflibercept was evaluated in the VEGF Trap-Eye: Investigation of Efficacy and Safety in Wet AMD (VIEW 1, VIEW 2) and showed noninferiority to ranibizumab.[37]

### Newer Anti–Vascular Endothelial Growth Factor Considerations

Brolucizumab is a single-chain antibody fragment that binds VEGF-A and was FDA approved for neovascular AMD in October 2019. The smaller molecular size is thought to penetrate tissue more effectively and clear more rapidly.[38] The HAWK and HARRIER trials compared brolucizumab with aflibercept and found that brolucizumab was noninferior for the treatment of neovascular macular degeneration. The safety of the drug is now being reevaluated because of serious postmarketing adverse events that have been reported, including inflammation and occlusive vasculitis with severe vision loss.[39]

The development of a port delivery system with ranibizumab is currently under investigation with promising results. The phase 3 Archway study examined the efficacy and safety of a surgically implanted port that can be refilled with ranibizumab in office every 6 months.[40,41] This option would significantly reduce the treatment burden of frequent injections, as many patients require treatment every 4 to 12 weeks with current options. The long-term evaluation of safety and efficacy is ongoing but shows promise in extending treatments up to 6 months.

### Current Practice

Practice patterns for patients with wet AMD are focused on a tailored approach based on physician and patient preferences, patient characteristics with extent of disease, and response to treatment.[34] Often if there is minimal or no response to 1 agent, the medication is switched to another. If patients maintain a good response to treatment, generally defined by improvement in vision and resolution of intraretinal and subretinal fluid, the interval for injection administration may be spaced out as tolerated. Generally spacing out of injection visits is done cautiously to ensure there is no recurrence. OCT imaging is critical to this algorithm of treatment to assess treatment response.

### Safety and Other Considerations

Although the associated risks of injections are considered low, there are certain local ocular adverse events and systemic events that need to be addressed with the patient before initiating treatment. Local ocular adverse events include elevated intraocular pressure, subconjunctival hemorrhage, vitreous hemorrhage, retinal detachment, and endophthalmitis. Endophthalmitis, an acute inflammatory response inside the eye usually due to infection, is one of the most dreaded complications following any intraocular procedure or surgery and may carry a poor visual prognosis. The risk of endophthalmitis following intravitreal injections for AMD is very low, with Daien and colleagues[42] reporting a rate of postinjection endophthalmitis of less than 1%.

The amount of systemic absorption of intravitreal anti-VEGF agents for patients with AMD is not fully understood. There is the theoretic risk of increased thrombotic events. Bressler and colleagues[43] reported an increased risk of stroke with higher doses of ranibizumab, although results were confounded by other variables and not considered significant. A large analysis of the systemic safety of ranibizumab in patients with neovascular AMD evaluated events such as myocardial infarction, cerebrovascular accident or transient ischemic attack, thromboembolic events, and major vascular events as per the Antiplatelet Trialists' Collaboration (APTC). The number of adverse events was low, which further supported the safety of the drug.[44] Kitchens and colleagues[45] found a similar safety profile for aflibercept with no statistically significant rate of major vascular events defined by APTC. Patients should be educated on the possible increased risk of thrombotic events, especially if there is a history of previous thrombotic events; however, the exact risk at this time is not fully understood. A promising large analysis of the risk of adverse advents after bevacizumab, ranibizumab, and aflibercept evaluated more than 80,000 patients and showed no increased risk of acute myocardial infarction, cerebral vascular disease, or major bleeding after administration of either of the 3 agents.[46]

Nephrotoxicity as a result of intravitreal injections is another potential systemic side effect with inconclusive results. Malignant hypertension, thrombotic microangiopathy, proteinuria, and nephrotic syndrome have been reported in patients with diabetes receiving intravitreal injections for diabetic retinopathy,[47] but there is little evidence to suggest a similar impact on patients who receive injections for AMD. These theoretic risks should be addressed with patients, especially in the presence of any underlying renal disease.

## PREVENTION AND LOW-VISION AIDS

The AREDS[48] established criteria for vitamin supplementation and demonstrated a 25% reduction in progression to advanced AMD. The current supplements consist of zinc, vitamin C, vitamin E, lutein, and zeaxanthin. The original formula included beta-carotene but because of the increased risk of lung cancer in smokers was replaced with lutein and zeaxanthin in the AREDS2 formulation (**Table 2**). Supplementation is recommended for intermediate AMD or those with early AMD in 1 eye and advanced AMD in the fellow eye but was not proven to be beneficial in patients with early AMD in both eyes. Supplementation is also not recommended for AMD prophylaxis or for those with a family history of AMD without the appropriate examination findings to support the qualifying diagnosis. Lifestyle

| Table 2 | |
| :--- | ---: |
| Age-Related Eye Disease Study2 nutrient supplementation and dosage | |
| Vitamin C | 400 mg |
| Vitamin E | 400 IU |
| Copper | 2 mg |
| Lutein | 10 mg |
| Zeaxanthin | 2 mg |
| Zinc | 80 mg |

modifications are advised for all patients and for those with early AMD in 1 or both eyes. Such modifications include dietary changes to incorporate antioxidant-rich foods and omega-3 and omega-6 fatty acids found in fish, along with weight loss and smoking cessation. Other modifiable risk factors include blood pressure and lipid control. There is conflicting evidence to support the role of UV light exposure and the development of AMD; however, limiting sun exposure is another potential lifestyle modification.[49]

### Low-Vision Aids

Access to low-vision aids is vital for patients with significant vision loss because of advanced AMD to optimize level of visual function for daily living. Previously, magnification lenses were the primary option available. Although these are an important tool, there are newer modalities available for those with low vision. The OrCam is a recently discovered optical recognition device that is mounted on a frame to assist with recognizing faces, text, and other objects.[50] In addition, smart devices now have many features that benefit those with low vision, such as enlarged font, brightness adjustment, dictation, and voice assist, to name a few.[51] Implantable miniature telescope technology is currently under investigation whereby eligible patients undergo a combined procedure with cataract extraction and telescope implantation.[51] These implants serve as a vision simulator and may be a promising option for the appropriate patient. A referral to a low-vision specialist for patients with vision loss owing to AMD or other eye disease can have a profound impact on improving a patient's ability to perform activities of daily living, as well as a positive impact in other nonocular aspects, such as fall risk and mental health.

### ON THE HORIZON

The current gold standard for the treatment of advanced AMD with anti-VEGF therapy requires frequent office visits and carries a significant treatment burden. Newer agents with other molecular targets are currently being investigated with the goal to enhance treatment efficacy and reduce burden of treatment. Faricimab is an angiopoietin-2 and VEGF-A inhibitor where phase 2 trials have shown a sustained response to treatment and may represent the opportunity to extend intervals between injections.[52] Conbercept binds to PLGF, VEGF-A, and VEGF-B and C and is approved for use in China.[53,54] The ongoing PANDA trials are designed to expand the sample size and compare global results.[55]

There are clinical trials currently underway for slowing the progression of geographic atrophy. The DERBY and OAKS trials are phase 3 studies evaluating the efficacy and safety of intravitreal pegcetacoplan, a complement component 3 inhibitor. Phase 2 results were promising and showed a reduced growth rate of geographic atrophy by 29% ($P = .008$) after 12 months.[56]

There is ongoing research in stem cell transplantation and gene replacement therapy focused on treating advanced disease. Clinical trials are underway for stem cell therapy focusing on the transplantation of RPE cells for tissue damaged by CNV or tissue loss owing to geographic atrophy.[57] There have been reports of success with improvement in vision. Early studies for gene therapy were discontinued because of unclear efficacy, but newer methods are on the horizon, and delivery strategies are being explored with promising results.[58]

Recent studies demonstrate a relationship between the use of Metformin for type 2 diabetes and a decreased risk of developing AMD.[59] Anti-inflammatory properties of the drug may play a role, and further investigations are underway.

## SUMMARY

AMD presents a major global health concern with a significant impact on quality of life for the elderly population. Loss of central vision impacts the ability to read, drive, recognize faces, and perform basic living tasks. There is significant variability in the phenotypic expression of the disease whereby early or intermediate AMD may cause minimal symptoms to advanced disease whereby the patient may experience visual distortion, decreased central visual acuity, scotomas, and total loss of central vision. The advent of anti-VEGF therapy has transformed visual outcomes for cases of advanced neovascular AMD. There are limited treatment options for those with advanced AMD secondary to geographic atrophy. Supplementation with AREDS2 vitamins can reduce risk of progression to advanced disease by 25% and is recommended for patients with advanced AMD in 1 eye and early or intermediate disease in the fellow eye. Risk factor modification includes smoking cessation, weight loss, lipid control, and incorporating antioxidant-rich foods into the diet.

## CLINICS CARE POINTS

- Age-related macular degeneration is primarily a disease of the elderly.
- Most patients have nonexudative or nonneovascular age-related macular degeneration and require ophthalmologic examinations and monitoring.
- Patients should be advised to quit smoking, control blood pressure and cholesterol levels, and maintain a healthy body mass index.
- Providers should be alerted to refer patients who complain of decreased vision, a central blind spot, or distortion in the vision for immediate ophthalmologic evaluation.
- Intravitreal injections are often necessary to preserve vision in those with advanced neovascular age-related macular degeneration.
- There is no treatment for advanced age-related macular degeneration because of geographic atrophy; however, ongoing trials are underway to slow the progression.
- The systemic side effects of intravitreal injections with anti–vascular endothelial growth factor agents may include thromboembolic events; however, these are theoretic risks with limited supporting evidence.

## DISCLOSURE

The authors have nothing to disclose.

## REFERENCES

1. Klein R, Klein BE, Knudtson MD, et al. Fifteen-year cumulative incidence of age-related macular degeneration: the Beaver Dam Eye Study. Ophthalmology 2007; 114(2):253–62.
2. Ferris FL III, Fine SL, Hyman L. Age-related macular degeneration and blindness due to neovascular maculopathy. Arch Ophthalmol 1984;102:1640–2.
3. Wong WL, Su X, Li X, et al. Global prevalence of age-related macular degeneration and disease burden projection for 2020 and 2040: a systematic review and meta-analysis. Lancet Glob Heal 2014;2:e106–16.
4. Casten RJ, Rovner BW. Update on depression and age-related macular degeneration. Curr Opin Ophthalmol 2013;24(3):239–43.

5. Age-related macular degeneration: facts & figures. BrightFocus Foundation; 2019. Available at: https://www.brightfocus.org/sources-macular-degeneration-facts-figures. Accessed June 6, 2020.

6. Chakravarthy U, Wong TY, Fletcher A, et al. Clinical risk factors for age-related macular degeneration: a systematic review and meta-analysis. BMC Ophthalmol 2010;10:31.

7. Davis MD, Gangnon RE, Lee LY, et al. Age-Related Eye Disease Study Group. The Age-Related Eye Disease Study severity scale for age-related macular degeneration: AREDS Report No. 17. Arch Ophthalmol 2005;123(11):1484–98 [Erratum in: Arch Ophthalmol. 2006;124(2):289-90].

8. Clemons TE, Milton RC, Klein R, et al. Age-related eye disease study research group. risk factors for the incidence of advanced age-related macular degeneration in the age-related eye disease study (AREDS) AREDS report no. 19. Ophthalmology 2005;112(4):533–9.

9. Velilla S, García-Medina JJ, García-Layana A, et al. Smoking and age-related macular degeneration: review and update. J Ophthalmol 2013;2013:895147.

10. Seddon JM, George S, Rosner B. Cigarette smoking, fish consumption, omega-3 fatty acid intake, and associations with age-related macular degeneration: the US Twin Study of Age-Related Macular Degeneration. Arch Ophthalmol 2006;124(7): 995–1001.

11. Joachim N, Mitchell P, Burlutsky G, et al. The incidence and progression of age-related macular degeneration over 15 years: the Blue Mountains Eye Study. Ophthalmology 2015;122(12):2482–9.

12. Vingerling JR, Hofman A, Grobbee DE, et al. Age-related macular degeneration and smoking. The Rotterdam Study. Arch Ophthalmol 1996;114(10):1193–6.

13. Pennington KL, DeAngelis MM. Epidemiology of age-related macular degeneration (AMD): associations with cardiovascular disease phenotypes and lipid factors. Eye Vis (Lond) 2016;3:34.

14. Comparison of Age-related Macular Degeneration Treatments Trials (CATT) Research Group, Maguire MG, Martin DF, Ying GS, et al. Five-year outcomes with anti-vascular endothelial growth factor treatment of neovascular age-related macular degeneration: the comparison of age-related macular degeneration treatments trials. Ophthalmology 2016;123(8):1751–61.

15. Varma R, Fraser-Bell S, Tan S, et al. Los Angeles Latino Eye Study Group. Prevalence of age-related macular degeneration in Latinos: the Los Angeles Latino Eye Study. Ophthalmology 2004;111(7):1288–97.

16. Parmet S, Lynm C, Glass RM. Age-related macular degeneration. JAMA 2006; 295(20):2438.

17. Abdelsalam A, Del Priore L, Zarbin MA. Drusen in age-related macular degeneration: pathogenesis, natural course, and laser photocoagulation-induced regression. Surv Ophthalmol 1999;44(1):1–29.

18. Klein R, Klein BE, Tomany SC, et al. Ten-year incidence and progression of age-related maculopathy: the Beaver Dam Eye Study. Ophthalmology 2002;109(10): 1767–79.

19. Ferris FL, Davis MD, Clemons TE, et al. A simplified severity scale for age-related macular degeneration: AREDS Report No. 18. Arch Ophthalmol 2005;123(11): 1570–4.

20. Fritsche LG, Fariss RN, Stambolian D, et al. Age-related macular degeneration: genetics and biology coming together. Annu Rev Genomics Hum Genet 2014; 15:151–71.

21. Gehrs KM, Anderson DH, Johnson LV, et al. Age-related macular degeneration–emerging pathogenetic and therapeutic concepts. Ann Med 2006;38(7):450–71.
22. Grunwald JE, Pistilli M, Daniel E, et al. Incidence and growth of geographic atrophy during 5 years of comparison of age-related macular degeneration treatments trials. Ophthalmology 2017;124(1):97–104.
23. Kiernan DF, Hariprasad SM, Rusu IM, et al. Epidemiology of the association between anticoagulants and intraocular hemorrhage in patients with neovascular age-related macular degeneration. Retina 2010;30(10):1573–8.
24. Sparrow JR, Hicks D, Hamel CP. The retinal pigment epithelium in health and disease. Curr Mol Med 2010;10(9):802–23.
25. Homayouni M. Vascular endothelial growth factors and their inhibitors in ocular neovascular disorders. J Ophthalmic Vis Res 2009;4(2):105–14.
26. Fritsche LG, Igl W, Bailey JN, et al. A large genome-wide association study of age-related macular degeneration highlights contributions of rare and common variants. Nat Genet 2016;48(2):134–43.
27. Csaky KG, Schachat AP, Kaiser PK, et al. The use of genetic testing in the management of patients with age-related macular degeneration: American Society of Retina Specialists Genetics Task Force Special Report. J VitreoRetinal Dis 2017; 1(1):75–8.
28. Gess AJ, Fung AE, Rodriguez JG. Imaging in neovascular age-related macular degeneration. Semin Ophthalmol 2011;26(3):225–33.
29. Fujimoto JG, Pitris C, Boppart SA, et al. Optical coherence tomography: an emerging technology for biomedical imaging and optical biopsy. Neoplasia 2000;2(1–2):9–25.
30. Ma J, Desai R, Nesper P, et al. Optical coherence tomographic angiography imaging in age-related macular degeneration. Ophthalmol Eye Dis 2017;9. 1179172116686075.
31. Jager RD, Mieler WF, Miller JW. Age-related macular degeneration. N Engl J Med 2008;358(24):2606–17 [Erratum in: N Engl J Med. 2008;359(16): 1736].
32. Lau PE, Jenkins KS, Layton CJ. Current evidence for the prevention of endophthalmitis in anti-VEGF intravitreal injections. J Ophthalmol 2018;2018:8567912.
33. Fallor MA, Simon SS, Gill MK, et al. Understanding patient perspectives of anti-VEGF treatment experience and effect in age-related macular degeneration. J Ophthalmol 2016;1(2):000111.
34. Brown D, Heier J, Boyer D, et al. Current best clinical practices-management of neovascular AMD. J VitreoRetinal Dis 2017;1(5):294–7.
35. Submacular Surgery Trials (SST) Research Group. Surgery for subfoveal choroidal neovascularization in age-related macular degeneration. Ophthalmology 2004;111(SST report no. 11):1967–80.
36. CATT Research Group. Ranibizumab and bevacizumab for neovascular age-related macular degeneration [published online April 28, 2011]. N Engl J Med 2011;364(20):1897–908.
37. Heier JS, Brown DM, Chong V, et al. Intravitreal aflibercept (VEGF trap-eye) in wet age-related macular degeneration. Ophthalmology 2012;119(12):2537–48 [published correction appears in Ophthalmology. 2013 Jan;120(1):209-10].
38. Gaudreault J, Gunde T, Floyd HS, et al. Preclinical pharmacology and safety of ESBA1008, a single-chain antibody fragment, investigated as potential treatment for age related macular degeneration. Invest Ophthalmol Vis Sci 2012;53:3025.
39. Hahn P, Arevalo JF, Blinder KJ, et al. Occlusive retinal vasculitis following intravitreal brolucizumab: an ASRS Research and Safety in Therapeutics (ReST) Committee Report. Retina Times 2020.

40. Pieramici D. LADDER trial of the Port Delivery System with ranibizumab: initial study results. Presented at the Retina Society 2018 annual meeting; San Francisco, California; September 14, 2018.
41. Pieramici D. Port Delivery System with ranibizumab (PDS): from dose ranging in LADDER phase 2 to ARCHWAY phase 3 study design. Presented at the 2018 American Academy of Ophthalmology Annual Meeting; Chicago, Illinois; October 27, 2018.
42. Daien V, Nguyen V, Essex RW, et al. Incidence and outcomes of infectious and noninfectious endophthalmitis after intravitreal injections for age-related macular degeneration. Ophthalmology 2018;125(1):66–74.
43. Bressler NM, Boyer DS, Williams DF, et al. Cerebrovascular accidents in patients treated for choroidal neovascularization with ranibizumab in randomized controlled trials. Retina 2012;32(9):1821–8.
44. Zarbin MA, Francom S, Grzeschik S, et al. Systemic safety in ranibizumab-treated patients with neovascular age-related macular degeneration: a patient-level pooled analysis. Ophthalmol Retina 2018;2:1087–96.
45. Kitchens JW, Do DV, Boyer DS, et al. Comprehensive review of ocular and systemic safety events with intravitreal aflibercept injection in randomized controlled trials. Ophthalmology 2016;123(7):1511–20.
46. Mahoney M, Payne S, Herrin J, et al. Risk of systemic adverse events after intravitreal bevacizumab, ranibizumab, and aflibercept in routine clinical practice. Ophthalmol 2020. https://doi.org/10.1016/j.ophtha.2020.07.062.
47. Hanna RM, Barsoum M, Arman F, et al. Nephrotoxicity induced by intravitreal vascular endothelial growth factor inhibitors: emerging evidence. Kidney Int 2019;96(3):572–80.
48. The Age-Related Eye Disease Study 2 (AREDS2) Research Group. Lutein + zeaxanthin and omega-3 fatty acids for age-related macular degeneration: the Age-Related Eye Disease Study 2 (AREDS2) randomized clinical trial. JAMA 2013;309(19):2005–15.
49. Zhou H, Zhang H, Yu A, et al. Association between sunlight exposure and risk of age-related macular degeneration: a meta-analysis. BMC Ophthalmol 2018; 18:331.
50. Moisseiev E, Mannis MJ. Evaluation of a portable artificial vision device among patients with low vision. JAMA Ophthalmol 2016;134(7):748–52.
51. Rush D. Helping patients maximize low-vision technology on smart devices. Retin Physician 2020;17:29–31.
52. Csaky KG. Data supporting the sustained efficacy of faricimab, a bispecific antibody neutralizing both angiopoietin-2 and VEGF-A. Presented at: American Academy of Ophthalmology annual meeting; Oct. 11-15, 2019; San Francisco.
53. Zhang M, Yu D, Yang C, et al. The pharmacology study of a new recombinant human VEGF receptor-fc fusion protein on experimental choroidal neovascularization. Pharm Res 2009;26(1):204–10.
54. Zhang M, Zhang J, Yan M, et al. Recombinant anti-vascular endothelial growth factor fusion protein efficiently suppresses choroidal neovascularization in monkeys. Mol Vis 2008;14:37–49.
55. Kirkner R. Pipeline Report: despite major approvals, the queue gets longer. Retina Specialist. Available at: https://www.retina-specialist.com/article/despite-major-approvals-the-queue-gets-longer. Accessed August 16, 2020.
56. Dole M. Apellis completes enrollment in two phase 3 studies of the targeted C3 therapy, pegcetacoplan, in patients with geographic atrophy (GA). Available at: https://

investors.apellis.com/news-releases/news-release-details/apellis-completes-enrollment-two-phase-3-studies-targeted-c3. Accessed August 16, 2020.

57. Zarbin M, Sugino I, Townes-Anderson E. Concise review: update on retinal pigment epithelium transplantation for age-related macular degeneration. Stem Cells Transl Med 2019. https://doi.org/10.1002/sctm.18-0282.

58. Ho A, Avery R. Gene therapy trials for wet age-related macular degeneration. Retina Today. Available at: https://retinatoday.com/articles/2019-may-june/gene-therapy-trials-for-wet-age-related-macular-degeneration. Accessed July 31, 2020.

59. Brown EE, Ball JD, Chen Z, et al. The common antidiabetic drug metformin reduces odds of developing age-related macular degeneration. Invest Ophthalmol Vis Sci 2019;60(5):1470–7.

# Glaucoma

Jessica Minjy Kang, MD, Angelo P. Tanna, MD*

## KEYWORDS

- Glaucoma • Open-angle glaucoma • Angle-closure glaucoma
- Secondary glaucoma • Glaucoma treatment

## KEY POINTS

- The term glaucoma refers to a group of conditions that have in common a progressive optic neuropathy characterized by optic disc excavation (cupping).
- Glaucoma is the leading cause of irreversible blindness worldwide.
- The most common type of glaucoma is primary open-angle glaucoma, a disease with a complex, multifactorial etiologic basis.
- Glaucoma is usually asymptomatic early in the disease.
- Intraocular pressure reduction is the only proven means of halting or slowing the progression of glaucoma. This pressure reduction can be accomplished with medical, laser, or surgical therapies.

## INTRODUCTION

Glaucoma is the leading cause of irreversible blindness worldwide.[1,2] The global prevalence of glaucoma in people aged 40 to 80 years is estimated to be 3.5%. With the growing number and proportion of older persons in the population, it is projected that 111.8 million people will have glaucoma in 2040.[3] Currently available treatments cannot reverse glaucomatous damage to the visual system; however, early diagnosis and treatment can prevent progression of the disease. In most cases, glaucoma is a chronic condition that requires lifelong management.

## PATHOPHYSIOLOGY

Glaucoma is a term that refers to a group of progressive optic neuropathies characterized by excavation or cupping of the optic disc, apoptotic degeneration of retinal

Conflicts of interest: J.M. Kang, None. A.P. Tanna, Bausch & Lomb (consultant); Ivantis (consultant); Zeiss (consultant).
Department of Ophthalmology, Northwestern University Feinberg School of Medicine, Chicago, IL, USA
* Corresponding author. Department of Ophthalmology, Northwestern University Feinberg School of Medicine, 645 North Michigan Avenue, Suite 440, Chicago, IL 60611.
E-mail address: atanna@northwestern.edu

ganglion cells, and corresponding vision loss. Retinal ganglion cells transmit visual information to the brain through axons, which comprise the optic nerve. The optic disc is the site where retinal ganglion cell axons coalesce, make a 90° turn, and pass through the sclera and lamina cribrosa (a highly organized, multilayered, fenestrated connective tissue populated with astrocytes) to exit the globe as the optic nerve (**Fig. 1**). The cup is the depression in the center of the optic disc. In glaucoma, progressive enlargement of the cup occurs because of damage to the lamina cribrosa and loss of retinal ganglion cell axons (**Fig. 2**).

Glaucoma is a multifactorial disease process, and its pathogenesis is incompletely understood. Although much attention is focused on the role of intraocular pressure (IOP), other factors such as abnormal ocular blood flow, abnormal structural susceptibility of the lamina cribrosa, low intracranial pressure, autoimmunity, and mitochondrial dysfunction may also be involved.[4]

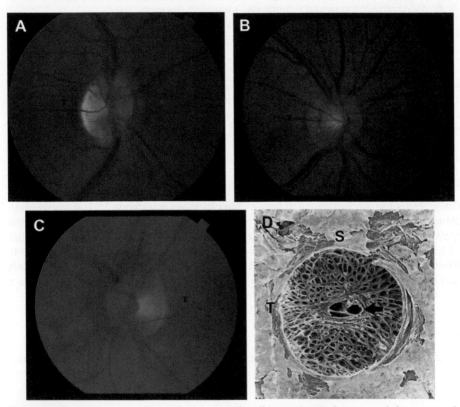

**Fig. 1.** (A–C) Healthy optic discs. (A) The central, yellow region is the cup and the surrounding pink tissue is the neural rim. The optic nerve is composed of the axons of retinal ganglion cells, most of which transmit visual information to the lateral geniculate nucleus. The striations visible in the retina are bundles of retinal ganglion cell axons in the retinal nerve fiber layer. The central retinal artery and vein enter the eye through the optic disc. (B) This normal optic disc has almost no discernible cup. (C) A normal left optic disc. (D) Scanning electron micrograph of the lamina cribrosa of the optic disc after trypsin digestion discloses a highly organized fenestrated network of connective tissue. The retinal ganglion cell axons traverse the lamina cribrosa where glial cells and capillaries support the neural tissue. The arrow marks the location of the central retina artery and vein. S, superior; T, temporal (lateral). ([D] *Courtesy of* Harry A. Quigley, M.D. Used with permission.)

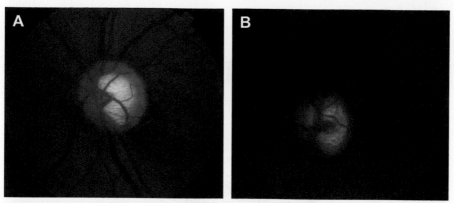

**Fig. 2.** (A,B) Examples of glaucomatous optic disc cupping. The optic disc cups are enlarged as a result of loss of neural rim tissue and lamina cribrosa damage. The pores of the lamina cribrosa are visible at the base of the cups.

Increased IOP is thought to damage the lamina cribrosa, resulting in loss of the normal structural and metabolic support of the retinal ganglion cell axons and impaired axoplasmic transport.[5,6] Decreased neurotrophic signaling to the retinal ganglion cells likely results in the initiation of apoptosis. IOP reduction is the only proven means to halt or slow the progression of glaucoma.

IOP is determined by the balance of aqueous humor production, aqueous humor outflow, and episcleral venous pressure. Aqueous humor is produced by the ciliary body and supports the metabolic processes of the avascular tissues in the anterior segment of the eye. Aqueous humor outflow takes place through 2 pathways originating in the anterior chamber angle: through the trabecular meshwork and Schlemm canal (conventional outflow), and through uveal tissues (unconventional outflow) (**Fig. 3**).

Tonometers used in clinical practice provide an estimate of IOP. Depending on the instrument used, IOP is determined by measuring the force required to flatten an area of the cornea, the amount of indentation of the cornea, or the deceleration of a probe rapidly projected onto the cornea. Many tonometers are available, including the Goldmann applanation tonometer, noncontact tonometers that use a column of air to flatten the cornea, rebound tonometers (ICare), and hand-held tonometers (Tono-Pen). Goldmann applanation tonometry is commonly used in clinical practice and in clinical trials (**Fig. 4**).

Although higher IOP plays a major role in glaucoma, it is not a defining criterion. Although the upper limit of normal IOP is often defined as 21 mm Hg, a large proportion of patients with glaucoma have an IOP lower than this, and not all patients with higher IOP (known as ocular hypertension) develop glaucoma.[7,8] As such, it is important to consider IOP as a continuous risk factor across the entire physiologic range.

Poor perfusion of the optic nerve may also contribute to disease development and progression.[9] Ocular perfusion pressure (OPP) is estimated in various ways. In general terms, it is the difference between systemic blood pressure and IOP. In population-based surveys, lower OPP has been identified as a risk factor for glaucoma and for the incident development of glaucoma.[10] Other studies have shown that lower OPP is an independent risk factor for worsening of the disease. Accordingly, for patients with severe glaucoma, overly aggressive treatment of systemic hypertension should be avoided.

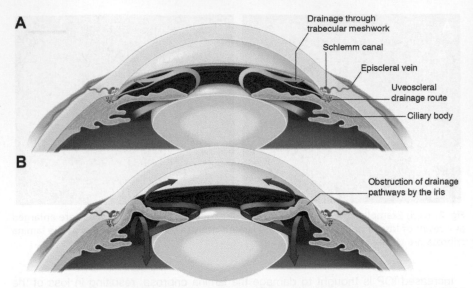

A
- Drainage through trabecular meshwork
- Schlemm canal
- Episcleral vein
- Uveoscleral drainage route
- Ciliary body

B
- Obstruction of drainage pathways by the iris

**Fig. 3.** Aqueous humor is produced by the ciliary body in the posterior chamber. This fluid then flows through the pupil into the anterior chamber. (*A*) Fluid can only exit the eye through structures in the anterior chamber (iridocorneal) angle. These structures are the trabecular meshwork (conventional outflow) and the ciliary body face (unconventional outflow). In most cases of open-angle glaucoma, increased resistance through the trabecular meshwork causes increase in IOP; however, no obstruction is clinically visible. (*B*) In primary angle closure, anatomic crowding of the iris and natural crystalline lens causes abnormal resistance of aqueous humor flow through the pupil. This pupillary block impairs the flow of aqueous humor through the pupil. Higher pressure posterior to the iris causes it to bow anteriorly into the iridocorneal angle and block the trabecular meshwork. (© 2021 American Academy of Ophthalmology; Used with permission.)

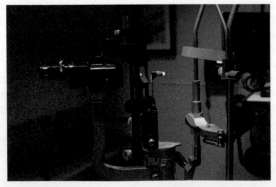

**Fig. 4.** The Goldmann applanation tonometer is widely regarded as the reference standard for clinical use. It measures the force (dynes) required to flatten a small area of the cornea, which is approximately equal to IOP/10 mm Hg. A topical anesthetic and fluorescent dye are required. While viewing the fluorescein-containing corneal tear film with the slit lamp microscope through a split-image prism, the examiner detects a visible end point that signifies corneal flattening.

## CLASSIFICATION

The glaucomas can be classified into open-angle glaucomas (OAGs) and angle-closure glaucomas (ACGs) to describe the anatomic status of the anterior chamber angle (**Table 1**). Each of these is further divided into primary or secondary, indicating the absence or presence, respectively, of other clinically identifiable ocular or systemic disorders to account for the glaucoma. The childhood glaucomas, such as primary congenital glaucoma and others associated with disorders of ocular development, are rare and are not discussed here.

The anterior chamber angle, or the iridocorneal angle, is the location of the trabecular meshwork and is a critically important region for aqueous humor outflow (see **Fig. 3**). The anatomic status of the angle (open or closed) is determined by ophthalmic examination.

Most eyes with glaucoma have increased resistance of outflow through the trabecular meshwork, which is usually associated with increased IOP. In eyes with open-angle glaucoma, this increase in resistance occurs in the absence of a clinically visible obstruction in the angle (see **Fig. 3**A). In contrast, angle closure refers to the anatomic configuration in which the peripheral iris is in contact with the trabecular meshwork, thereby obstructing outflow of aqueous humor. The most common mechanism by which angle closure occurs is pupillary block, a condition in which abnormally tight contact between the iris and lens can cause increased resistance of aqueous flow through the pupil. This condition results in a pressure gradient that causes the iris to bow forward and obstruct the trabecular meshwork (see **Fig. 3**B). Pupillary block is most common in hyperopic (far-sighted) eyes that have more crowded anterior segments.

**Table 1**
**Glaucoma classification and selected examples**

| Open-Angle Glaucoma | Angle-Closure Glaucomas | Childhood Glaucomas |
|---|---|---|
| Primary open-angle glaucoma<br>Secondary OAGs<br>• Pigmentary glaucoma<br>• Pseudoexfoliation glaucoma<br>• Uveitic glaucoma (can also have a combined, angle-closure mechanism)<br>• Steroid-induced glaucoma<br>• Traumatic glaucoma<br>• Glaucoma associated with increased episcleral venous pressure (eg, carotid-cavernous fistula, cavernous sinus thrombosis, thyroid eye disease) | Primary angle-closure glaucoma<br>• Pupillary block<br>• Plateau iris<br>Secondary angle-closure glaucoma<br>• Medication induced<br>• Lens induced<br>• Neovascular<br>• Iridocorneal endothelial syndrome<br>• Ciliary body or iris cyst or tumor | Primary congenital glaucoma<br>Juvenile open-angle glaucoma<br>Glaucoma following (congenital) cataract surgery<br>Glaucoma associated with nonacquired systemic anomalies<br>• Axenfeld-Rieger syndrome<br>• Peters anomaly<br>• Aniridia<br>Glaucoma associated with nonacquired systemic disease<br>• Chromosomal disorders<br>• Connective tissue disorders<br>• Metabolic disorders<br>• Neurofibromatosis<br>• Sturge-Weber syndrome<br>• Congenital rubella |

Primary OAG (POAG) and primary ACG (PACG) are the two most common forms of glaucoma. It is estimated that the number of people blind from glaucoma in 2020 globally is 11.1 million.[11] Disease burdens of POAG and PACG differ based on geographic regions and ethnic groups. POAG prevalence is highest among blacks and Hispanic people, and PACG is most prevalent among Asian and Inuit people.[3]

Excluding the childhood glaucomas, more than 60 forms of secondary glaucoma have been described. These forms can occur because of numerous underlying mechanisms, including trauma, intraocular bleeding, neoplasia, inflammation, neovascularization retinal ischemia, and exposure to a variety of medications (see **Table 1**).

## SYMPTOMS

Glaucoma usually progresses slowly, and thus patients often remain asymptomatic until the disease is severe. Population-based surveys suggest around 50% of people with glaucoma are unaware of their diagnosis, even in developed nations.[12–14] Severe, acute IOP increase usually results in pain and decreased vision. Moderately increased IOP, which is much more common in glaucoma, is usually imperceptible to the patient.

When patients are symptomatic, the description of glaucomatous vision loss as tunnel vision is a commonly held misconception.[15] Except in very advanced disease, areas of glaucomatous visual field loss are commonly described by patients as blurred areas, not absolute scotomas. As the damage becomes severe, patients describe their vision as diffusely foggy or dark. In late stages, glaucoma may progress to total loss of light perception.[16]

## DIAGNOSTIC EVALUATION

Because glaucomatous vision loss is irreversible, early diagnosis and treatment is essential to prevent morbidity. Screening and identification of high-risk patients by ophthalmologists allows the early detection of glaucoma. All adults more than the age of 40 years should have examinations to screen for various disease processes, including glaucoma.[17]

### Examination

The complete and accurate diagnosis of glaucoma requires a thorough ophthalmic examination. Glaucomatous optic disc damage, excavation or cupping, can be visualized with ophthalmoscopy (see **Fig. 2**).[18,19] Because glaucomatous damage typically occurs in the inferotemporal and superotemporal regions of the optic nerve, a larger vertical compared with horizontal cup-to-disc ratio may be observed, with the cup often extending abnormally close to the inferior or superior border of the optic disc.[20]

Early diagnosis of glaucoma may be challenging because there is wide variation in the appearance of the healthy optic nerve and overlap in the clinical appearance of the optic nerve among some normal eyes and some eyes with glaucoma. Diagnosis often requires longitudinal evaluation and documentation of structural change in the optic nerve of persons suspected of having early glaucoma.

Physicians other than ophthalmologists may be able to detect glaucomatous optic disc damage with direct ophthalmoscopy; however, the view through an undilated pupil is often poor and the absence of a stereoscopic view severely limits the clinician's ability to accurately detect optic disc excavation.

### Imaging

Photographs can be useful for monitoring the appearance of the optic disc and detecting pathologic change over time. The advent of optical coherence tomography (OCT) has revolutionized the ability to monitor the anatomic structures affected by glaucoma. OCT is a noninvasive imaging technique that relies on the use of Michelson interferometry to decode the interference patterns of light reflected from intraocular tissues. It allows quantitative measurement of the optic nerve, the retinal ganglion cell axon layer (known as the retinal nerve fiber layer), and the layer of the retinal ganglion cell bodies (**Fig. 5**). Structural changes such as retinal nerve fiber layer thinning typically occur before the development of functional losses detectable by conventional visual field testing.[21]

### Perimetry

Formal testing to evaluate the central and midperipheral portions of the visual field is important for the diagnosis and management of glaucoma. The goal of testing is to determine the minimum intensity of light stimuli detectable at locations in the central 30° of the visual field at 6° intervals.

Characteristic patterns of glaucomatous visual field damage correspond with the location of injury to retinal ganglion cell axon bundles at the level of the lamina cribrosa. The location of injury coupled with the anatomic organization of the axon bundles results in visual field defects that typically respect the horizontal midline early in the disease (**Fig. 6**). In contrast, defects respecting the vertical midline indicate central neurologic lesions.[22]

## GENETICS

Although certain types of developmental glaucomas are mendelian disorders, most cases of POAG and PACG result from a complex interaction of genetic and

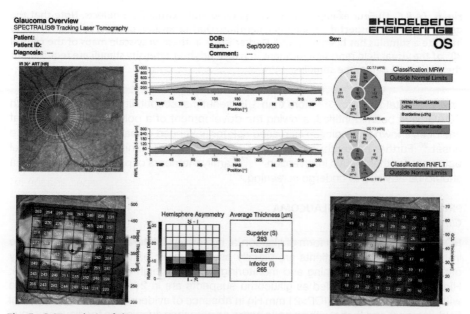

**Fig. 5.** OCT analysis of the posterior segment of an eye with glaucoma. The neural rim thickness, retinal nerve fiber layer thickness, and macular thickness are all decreased because of glaucoma damage. Serial testing can be performed to monitor neural tissue thickness for change over time.

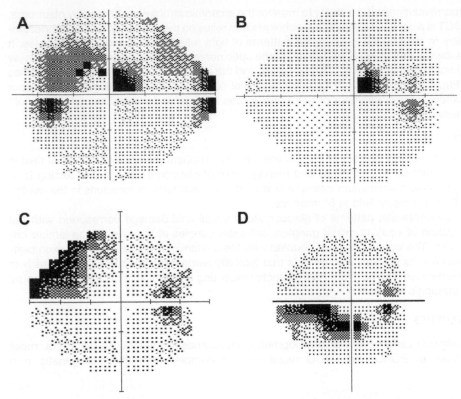

**Fig. 6.** (A,B,C, D) Four examples of typical glaucomatous visual field defects. Note that the defects generally respect the horizontal meridian. During testing, patients press a button to indicate a stimulus has been observed. Darker areas in these gray-scale maps of the central 30° of the visual field represent locations in which brighter-intensity stimuli are required for the patient to detect the stimulus.

environmental factors.[23–25] More than 100 genetic susceptibility loci associated with POAG have been identified, allowing the development of a polygenic risk score that has been shown to predict an increased risk for advanced disease and earlier disease onset.[26] Further research is needed to refine genetic screening and identify novel pathways for therapeutic intervention.[23,27] Family members of patients with glaucoma should be advised to undergo screening.

## PRIMARY OPEN-ANGLE GLAUCOMA
### Clinical Diagnosis

POAG, the most common form of glaucoma, is typically bilateral but often asymmetric in severity.[3] Because patients are usually asymptomatic early in the disease, early detection requires screening and monitoring of certain high-risk patients (**Table 2**). High-risk patients classified as glaucoma suspects are in 2 major categories: those with ocular hypertension (IOP>21 mm Hg in absence of evidence of optic disc or visual field damage) and those with an optic nerve appearance suspicious for glaucomatous damage.[30] Such patients should be examined by an ophthalmologist at least annually to monitor for evidence of conversion to definite POAG from progressive structural (optic disc or retinal nerve fiber layer) or functional (visual field) damage.[30] Some

**Table 2**
**Selected risk factors for glaucoma**

| Primary Open-Angle Glaucoma[28] | Primary Angle-Closure Glaucoma[29] |
|---|---|
| • Older age | • Older age |
| • Increased IOP | • Family history of angle closure |
| • Family history of glaucoma | • Asian or Inuit descent |
| • African race or Latino/Hispanic ethnicity | • Hyperopia (far-sightedness) |
| • Myopia (near-sightedness) | • Female sex |

patients with ocular hypertension with high-risk characteristics may be treated with medication or laser to decrease the IOP in order to reduce the risk of the development of POAG.

## PRIMARY ANGLE CLOSURE
### Clinical Diagnosis

Some patients with narrow anterior chamber angles develop primary angle closure, the term used to describe the presence of adhesions of the iris to the trabecular meshwork and/or ocular hypertension without glaucomatous optic nerve damage. Over time, some patients with primary angle closure go on to develop primary angle-closure glaucoma, the distinguishing characteristic being the presence of optic nerve damage.

Usually, primary angle closure is a chronic, asymptomatic process. Uncommonly, patients with narrow angles can present with acute primary angle-closure crisis. In this condition, deep eye pain, headache, blurred vision, halos or rainbows around lights, eye redness, and nausea occur as a result of sudden and severe IOP increase triggered by pupillary block.

Risk factors for primary angle closure include ocular features that are associated with crowding of the anterior segment, such as hyperopia (far-sightedness), as well as older age and a family history of the disease.[31] The condition is more prevalent in women and patients of Asian or Inuit descent.[32] Laser iridotomy may be performed prophylactically in some patients with narrow angles in the absence of other disease-associated features.

## SECONDARY GLAUCOMAS

Secondary glaucomas encompass a broad spectrum of diseases. By definition, they have a clinically identifiable cause for IOP increase. Some examples of secondary glaucomas are discussed here.

### Pseudoexfoliation Glaucoma

Pseudoexfoliation glaucoma is the most common secondary glaucoma.[33] Abnormal extracellular matrix material in the outflow pathway leads to IOP increase.[34] Pseudoexfoliation syndrome is a systemic disorder of the extracellular matrix that has several ocular consequences and has also been shown to be associated with an increased risk of pelvic organ prolapse and inguinal hernia. It is clinically characterized by the presence of abnormal fibrillar deposits on the surface of the lens and iris that can be detected by examination with slit lamp biomicroscopy (**Fig. 7**). The condition is rare in patients less than 65 years of age. The prevalence is 5% among persons 75 to 85 years of age in the United States and as high as 25% in Scandinavia. A genome-wide association study led to the discovery of a strong association with

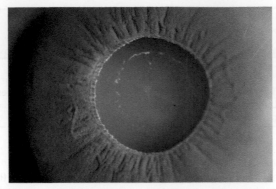

**Fig. 7.** Pseudoexfoliation syndrome. Abnormal fibrillar deposits of elastin and collagen on the surface of the lens and pupil border. The condition is commonly associated with the development of increased IOP and secondary open-angle glaucoma.

variants of *LOXL1* (lysyl oxidase–1); these were present in greater than 99% of affected individuals and ~80% of controls.[35] The abnormal fibrillar material is thought to arise as a result of abnormal maintenance of elastin and collagen. Other genetic and environmental factors, such as ocular ultraviolet light exposure, likely play a strong role in the development of this disorder.[36,37]

### Neovascular Glaucoma

Conditions such as diabetic retinopathy, retinal vascular occlusions, and carotid artery obstructive disease can lead to retinal ischemia with a resultant release of proangiogenic factors such as vascular endothelial growth factor (VEGF). Neovascularization can then develop in the anterior segment of the eye and over the iridocorneal angle, obstructing aqueous humor outflow.

Patients usually present with symptomatic, acute IOP increase. A 2-pronged treatment strategy is used. Retinal laser photocoagulation and intraocular injections of anti-VEGF agents are used to induce regression of the neovascular tissue, and medical and surgical therapy are used to decrease the IOP. Although many patients do well with modern therapy, some patients experience severe vision loss, often because of the underlying cause for the retinal ischemia. Patients with neovascular glaucoma require optimization of their underlying vasculopathic risk factors to mitigate the risk of additional vascular events.

### Steroid-Responsive Ocular Hypertension

Chronic corticosteroid therapy may, in some individuals, result in increased resistance to outflow through the trabecular meshwork and thereby cause IOP increase. Although this is most common with ophthalmic or oral steroid therapy, it can occur with steroid administration through any route (eg, nasal, inhaled, dermatologic, and intra-articular).[38] IOP can increase after 2 weeks of treatment and is typically reversible after cessation of steroid exposure.[39]

### Medication-Induced Angle Closure

Medications may induce unilateral or bilateral acute angle closure by 2 different mechanisms (**Table 3**).[41] The first, pupillary block, is most likely to occur when the pupil is in a mid-dilated state. In susceptible patients with narrow angles, agents that can cause subtle pupil dilatation, such as adrenergic agonists and anticholinergic drugs, may trigger an acute angle-closure crisis. The second is an idiosyncratic reaction in which

**Table 3**
**Medications that may cause acute angle closure**

| Drug Class | Drug |
| --- | --- |
| Adrenergic drugs | Phenylephrine (ophthalmic)<br>Naphazoline (intranasal)<br>Salbutamol (inhaled) |
| Anticholinergic drugs | Atropine (ophthalmic)<br>Oxybutynin<br>Scopolamine<br>Botulinum toxin (intramuscular) |
| Antidepressant drugs | Venlafaxine<br>Escitalopram<br>Bupropion |
| Sulfonamide drugs | Topiramate<br>Acetazolamide[a]<br>Methazolamide[a] |

[a] Carbonic anhydrase inhibitors such as acetazolamide and methazolamide are still indicated for use as IOP-lowering agents and angle closure caused by exposure to these medications is rare.[40]

sulfonamide agents, most commonly topiramate and carbonic anhydrase inhibitors, cause edema of the ciliary body leading to forward displacement of the lens and iris and bilateral angle closure. Rapid identification and removal of the offending agent, medical therapy to decrease the IOP, and systemic corticosteroids can help decrease the risk of vision loss.

## TREATMENT

IOP reduction is the only proven means of halting or slowing the progression of glaucoma.[8,28,42–44] Even patients with POAG in whom baseline IOP is less than or equal to 21 mm Hg benefit from treatment to further decrease the IOP.[45] First-line treatment is typically either a topical IOP-lowering medication or laser trabeculoplasty (discussed later).[46]

In primary angle-closure disease, pupillary block must also be addressed. In addition to IOP-lowering medications, iridotomy or lens extraction is required.[47]

Treatment of severe, acute IOP increase of any cause can usually be accomplished with topical and oral medications, sometimes in combination with systemic hyperosmotic agents such as mannitol or glycerin. When the underlying cause is pupillary block, iridotomy or lens extraction should then be performed as soon as possible. Although acute angle-closure crisis is typically unilateral, about half of fellow eyes can develop an acute crisis within 5 years, necessitating prophylactic iridotomy or lens extraction.[29,48] Unlike most cataract surgery, which is performed with the aim of improving vision, the primary goal of lens extraction for angle closure is to open the iridocorneal angle by replacing the large natural lens with a thin artificial lens.

### Medical Therapy

Topical glaucoma medications decrease IOP by reducing aqueous humor production or improving outflow (**Table 4**). The most frequently used medication class is the prostaglandin $F_{2\alpha}$ analogues. These agents activate matrix metalloproteases, which degrade collagen in the ciliary body, allowing increased outflow of aqueous humor directly through this tissue (unconventional outflow). Approximately half of patients require 2 or more medications to adequately decrease their IOP.[50]

**Table 4**
**Topical glaucoma medications**

| Class | Mechanism | Side Effects | Contraindications/ Considerations |
|---|---|---|---|
| Prostaglandin $F_{2\alpha}$ Analogue (teal cap)<br>• Latanoprost<br>• Travoprost<br>• Bimatoprost<br>• Tafluprost | ↑ AH outflow | Iris and periocular skin color change (irreversible), eyelash growth, conjunctival hyperemia | Active uveitis |
| Rho kinase inhibitor (white cap)<br>• Netarsudil | ↑ AH outflow<br>↓ EVP | Conjunctival hyperemia and hemorrhages, pain, blurred vision | — |
| β-Blocker (yellow cap)<br>• Timolol<br>• Levobunolol<br>• Caretolol<br>• Betaxolol ($\beta_1$ selective) | ↓ AH production | Bradycardia, bronchospasm, hypotension, reduced exercise tolerance<br>Betaxolol with lower risk of pulmonary side effects | Asthma/COPD, severe CHF, second-degree or third-degree AV block, bradycardia<br>Less effective in those already on high-dose systemic β-blocker |
| Alpha₂ agonist (purple cap)<br>• Brimonidine<br>• Apraclonidine | ↓ AH production<br>↑ AH outflow | Conjunctivitis, dry mouth, fatigue, systemic hypotension | Infants and children |
| Carbonic anhydrase inhibitor (orange cap)<br>• Dorzolamide<br>• Brinzolamide | ↓ AH production | Ocular irritation, allergic dermatitis, metallic taste, corneal edema | Sickle cell disease<br>Caution in patients with sulfa allergy, although may be considered[49] |
| Cholinergic agonist (green cap)<br>• Pilocarpine | ↑ AH outflow | Blurred vision, difficulty with night vision, headache, paradoxic angle closure, retinal tear | Ocular inflammation |

*Abbreviations:* AH, aqueous humor; AV, arteriovenous; CHF, congestive heart failure, COPD, chronic obstructive pulmonary disease; EVP, episcleral venous pressure.

Systemic absorption of topically administered ophthalmic medications occurs through the nasolacrimal drainage system. Because of the absence of first-pass hepatic metabolism, serum levels can reach those achieved with oral administration of, for example, timolol. This condition can lead to serious adverse events, particularly associated with the use of topical β-blockers and alpha₂-adrenergic agonists. Eyelid closure and nasolacrimal occlusion (application of digital pressure to the region over the nasolacrimal sac) can enhance intraocular penetration of medications and reduce systemic absorption.[51]

### Laser Surgery

### Laser trabeculoplasty
Laser trabeculoplasty is a procedure in which laser energy is applied to the trabecular meshwork with a resultant reduction in the resistance to aqueous outflow. Although the mechanism is incompletely understood, it likely involves the recruitment of monocytes and replication of pigmented endothelial cells in the trabecular meshwork.[52]

### Laser peripheral iridotomy

Laser peripheral iridotomy (LPI) can be performed for angle closure with pupillary block. Laser energy is used to create a small hole in the peripheral iris, allowing aqueous humor to bypass the pupil. After an LPI, many patients have persistently increased IOP and require additional treatment.[53]

### Incisional glaucoma surgery

In patients with inadequately controlled IOP despite medical and laser therapy, a variety of incisional surgery approaches may be used. In addition, initial surgical therapy may be considered for patients who present with advanced disease.

Glaucoma surgeries include procedures designed to either reduce resistance to aqueous humor outflow in the conventional pathway or create a new pathway for aqueous humor outflow. The former category is known as minimally invasive glaucoma surgery (MIGS) and typically involves implantation of a microstent allowing bypass of the trabecular meshwork or scaffolding of the Schlemm canal. Alternatively, the trabecular meshwork can be incised or disrupted. These procedures are often performed in conjunction with cataract surgery and usually have a safety profile similar to that of cataract surgery alone.[54] The magnitude of IOP reduction is often modest; therefore, these procedures are typically indicated for patients with mild to moderate glaucoma damage.[55]

Glaucoma tube shunt surgery and trabeculectomy are fistulizing procedures that involve the creation a new outflow track for aqueous humor to the subconjunctival space, and typically result in larger magnitudes of IOP reduction compared with MIGS.

Glaucoma tube shunt surgery involves implanting a tube in the eye that shunts aqueous to a silicone plate located at the equator of the globe, around which aqueous can diffuse into surrounding extraocular tissues (**Fig. 8**). In trabeculectomy surgery, a scleral flap is created, underneath which an ostium into the anterior chamber is created (**Fig. 9**). Aqueous humor flows through the ostium and scleral flap, into the subconjunctival space, forming a bleb, which is an aqueous humor–filled elevation of the conjunctiva under the upper eyelid. Despite the use of local antifibrotic therapy

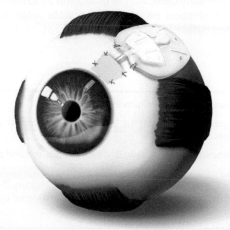

**Fig. 8.** Glaucoma tube shunt surgery. Drainage devices can be used to provide an alternative path for aqueous outflow and IOP reduction. A tube is inserted into the anterior chamber of the eye and is connected to a plate that is placed underneath the conjunctiva and serves as a spacer around which aqueous humor can diffuse into extraocular tissues. The entire device is made of silicone. (Figure courtesy of the New World Medical. Used with permission.)

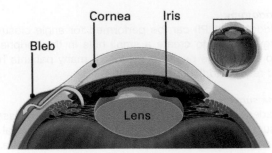

**Fig. 9.** In trabeculectomy, an ostium into the anterior chamber is fashioned under a scleral flap located under the upper eyelid. This ostium allows aqueous humor to exit the eye in a controlled fashion. Aqueous humor accumulates under the conjunctiva, forming an area of elevation called a bleb. (Courtesy of the American Academy of Ophthalmology. Used with permission.)

at the time of surgery, the formation of subconjunctival fibrotic tissue can result in subsequent failure.

The risk of adverse events associated with these procedures is substantial; therefore, these procedures are typically only performed in patients at high risk of symptomatic progression of their disease. Because a direct pathway between the subconjunctival space and intraocular structures is created, there is an ongoing risk of intraocular infection ranging from 0.5% over 5 years for tube shunt surgery to 1.5% to 2% for trabeculectomy. Symptoms or signs of infection, including redness, photophobia, pain, and vision loss, should be urgently evaluated by an ophthalmologist.[56,57]

## DISCUSSION AND SUMMARY

Although irreversible, glaucomatous damage can be halted or slowed with early detection and appropriate treatment. At present, the only proven means of treatment is IOP reduction with medications, laser treatment, and incisional surgery. Physicians can play a significant role in the early detection of glaucoma by identifying risk factors and optic disc cupping on examination, referring appropriate patients for ophthalmic consultation, and by educating patients that glaucoma requires medication adherence and regular follow-up.

## CLINICS CARE POINTS

- Glaucoma is the leading cause of irreversible blindness worldwide.[3]
- Because of the slowly progressive nature of the disease process, almost all patients are asymptomatic until late stages of the disease.
- Acute angle-closure crisis, although rare, results in decreased vision, eye and periorbital pain, eye redness, and nausea.[32]
- Risk factors for both POAG and PACG include older age and family history.[28,29] Patients with glaucoma should be reminded to advise family members to be evaluated by an ophthalmologist.

## ACKNOWLEDGMENTS

The authors gratefully acknowledge Kaitlyn M. Veto for her expertise in obtaining the clinical photographs used in this article.

## REFERENCES

1. Flaxman SR, Bourne RRA, Resnikoff S, et al. Global causes of blindness and distance vision impairment 1990-2020: a systematic review and meta-analysis. Lancet Glob Health 2017;5(12):e1221–34.
2. Kingman S. Glaucoma is second leading cause of blindness globally. Bull World Health Organ 2004;82(11):887–8.
3. Tham YC, Li X, Wong TY, et al. Global prevalence of glaucoma and projections of glaucoma burden through 2040: a systematic review and meta-analysis. Ophthalmology 2014;121(11):2081–90.
4. Quigley HA. Glaucoma. Lancet 2011;377(9774):1367–77.
5. Gaasterland DE, Pollack IP. Initial experience with a new method of laser transscleral cyclophotocoagulation for ciliary ablation in severe glaucoma. Trans Am Ophthalmol Soc 1992;90:225–46.
6. Burgoyne CF, Crawford Downs J, Bellezza AJ, et al. The optic nerve head as a biomechanical structure: a new paradigm for understanding the role of IOP-related stress and strain in the pathophysiology of glaucomatous optic nerve head damage. Prog Retin Eye Res 2005;24(1):39–73.
7. Lichter PR, Musch DC, Gillespie BW, et al. Interim clinical outcomes in the Collaborative Initial Glaucoma Treatment Study comparing initial treatment randomized to medications or surgery. Ophthalmology 2001;108(11): 1943–53.
8. Kass MA, Heuer DK, Higginbotham EJ, et al. The Ocular Hypertension Treatment Study: a randomized trial determines that topical ocular hypotensive medication delays or prevents the onset of primary open-angle glaucoma. Arch Ophthalmol 2002;120(6):701–13 [discussion: 829–30].
9. Leske MC. Ocular perfusion pressure and glaucoma: clinical trial and epidemiologic findings. Curr Opin Ophthalmol 2009;20(2):73–8.
10. Khawaja AP, Crabb DP, Jansonius NM. The role of ocular perfusion pressure in glaucoma cannot be studied with multivariable regression analysis applied to surrogates. Invest Ophthalmol Vis Sci 2013;54(7):4619–20.
11. Quigley HA, Broman AT. The number of people with glaucoma worldwide in 2010 and 2020. Br J Ophthalmol 2006;90(3):262–7.
12. Leite MT, Sakata LM, Medeiros FA. Managing glaucoma in developing countries. Arq Bras Oftalmol 2011;74(2):83–4.
13. Hennis A, Wu SY, Nemesure B, et al. Awareness of incident open-angle glaucoma in a population study: the Barbados Eye Studies. Ophthalmology 2007;114(10): 1816–21.
14. Budenz DL, Barton K, Whiteside-de Vos J, et al. Prevalence of glaucoma in an urban West African population: the Tema Eye Survey. JAMA Ophthalmol 2013; 131(5):651–8.
15. Hu CX, Zangalli C, Hsieh M, et al. What Do Patients With Glaucoma See? Visual Symptoms Reported by Patients With Glaucoma. Am J Med Sci 2014;348(5): 403–9.
16. Pickett JE, Terry SA, O'Connor PS, et al. Early loss of central visual acuity in glaucoma. Ophthalmology 1985;92(7):891–6.
17. Turbert D. Get an eye disease screening at 40 2019. Available at: https://www.aao.org/eye-health/tips-prevention/screening. Accessed Aug 28, 2020.
18. Quigley HA. Open-Angle Glaucoma. N Engl J Med 1993;328(15):1097–106.

19. Quigley HA, Addicks EM, Green WR, et al. Optic nerve damage in human glaucoma. II. The site of injury and susceptibility to damage. Arch Ophthalmol 1981; 99(4):635–49.
20. Jonas JB, Fernández MC, Stürmer J. Pattern of glaucomatous neuroretinal rim loss. Ophthalmology 1993;100(1):63–8.
21. Alasil T, Wang K, Yu F, et al. Correlation of retinal nerve fiber layer thickness and visual fields in glaucoma: a broken stick model. Am J Ophthalmol 2014;157(5): 953–9.
22. Gilpin LB, Steward WC, Shields MB, et al. Hemianopic offsets in the visual field of patients with glaucoma. Graefes Arch Clin Exp Ophthalmol 1990;228(5):450–3.
23. Wiggs JL, Pasquale LR. Genetics of glaucoma. Hum Mol Genet 2017;26(R1): R21–7. https://doi.org/10.1093/hmg/ddx184. PMID: 28505344; PMCID: PMC6074793.
24. Khor CC, Do T, Jia H, et al. Genome-wide association study identifies five new susceptibility loci for primary angle closure glaucoma. Nat Genet 2016;48(5): 556–62.
25. Vithana EN, Khor C-C, Qiao C, et al. Genome-wide association analyses identify three new susceptibility loci for primary angle closure glaucoma. Nat Genet 2012; 44(10):1142–6.
26. Craig JE, Han X, Qassim A, et al. Multitrait analysis of glaucoma identifies new risk loci and enables polygenic prediction of disease susceptibility and progression. Nat Genet 2020;52(2):160–6.
27. Liu C, Nongpiur ME, Khor C-C, et al. Primary angle closure glaucoma genomic associations and disease mechanism. Curr Opin Ophthalmol 2020;31(2).
28. Prum BE Jr, Rosenberg LF, Gedde SJ, et al. Primary open-angle glaucoma preferred practice pattern® guidelines. Ophthalmology 2016;123(1):P41–111.
29. Prum BE Jr, Herndon LW Jr, Moroi SE, et al. Primary angle closure preferred practice pattern® guidelines. Ophthalmology 2016;123(1):P1–40.
30. Prum BE Jr, Lim MC, Mansberger SL, et al. Primary open-angle glaucoma suspect preferred practice pattern® guidelines. Ophthalmology 2016;123(1): P112–51.
31. Ahram DF, Alward WL, Kuehn MH. The genetic mechanisms of primary angle closure glaucoma. Eye (London, England) 2015;29(10):1251–9.
32. Yip JL, Foster PJ. Ethnic differences in primary angle-closure glaucoma. Curr Opin Ophthalmol 2006;17(2):175–80.
33. Ritch R. Exfoliation syndrome-the most common identifiable cause of open-angle glaucoma. J Glaucoma 1994;3(2):176–7.
34. Schlötzer-Schrehardt U, Naumann GOH. Ocular and systemic pseudoexfoliation syndrome. Am J Ophthalmol 2006;141(5):921–37.e2.
35. Thorleifsson G, Magnusson KP, Sulem P, et al. Common sequence variants in the LOXL1 gene confer susceptibility to exfoliation glaucoma. Science 2007; 317(5843):1397–400.
36. Jiwani AZ, Pasquale LR. Exfoliation syndrome and solar exposure: new epidemiological insights into the pathophysiology of the disease. Int Ophthalmol Clin 2015;55(4):13–22.
37. Pasquale LR, Kang JH, Wiggs JL. Prospects for gene-environment interactions in exfoliation syndrome. J Glaucoma 2014;23(8 Suppl 1):S64–7.
38. Roberti G, Oddone F, Agnifili L, et al. Steroid-induced glaucoma: Epidemiology, pathophysiology, and clinical management. Surv Ophthalmol 2020;65(4): 458–72. https://doi.org/10.1016/j.survophthal.2020.01.002. Epub 2020 Feb 11. PMID: 32057761.

39. Phulke S, Kaushik S, Kaur S, et al. Steroid-induced Glaucoma: An Avoidable Irreversible Blindness. J Curr Glaucoma Pract 2017;11(2):67–72. https://doi.org/10.5005/jp-journals-l0028-1226. Epub 2017 Aug 5. PMID: 28924342; PMCID: PMC5577123.

40. Murphy RM, Bakir B, O'Brien C, et al. Drug-induced bilateral secondary angle-closure glaucoma: a literature synthesis. J Glaucoma 2016;25(2):e99–105.

41. Lachkar Y, Bouassida W. Drug-induced acute angle closure glaucoma. Curr Opin Ophthalmol 2007;18(2):129–33.

42. Leske MC, Heijl A, Hussein M, et al. Factors for glaucoma progression and the effect of treatment: the early manifest glaucoma trial. Arch Ophthalmol 2003; 121(1):48–56.

43. The Advanced Glaucoma Intervention Study (AGIS): 7. The relationship between control of intraocular pressure and visual field deterioration. The AGIS Investigators. Am J Ophthalmol 2000;130(4):429–40.

44. Garway-Heath DF, Crabb DP, Bunce C, et al. Latanoprost for open-angle glaucoma (UKGTS): a randomised, multicentre, placebo-controlled trial. Lancet 2015;385(9975):1295–304.

45. Comparison of glaucomatous progression between untreated patients with normal-tension glaucoma and patients with therapeutically reduced intraocular pressures. Collaborative Normal-Tension Glaucoma Study Group. Am J Ophthalmol 1998;126(4):487–97.

46. Gazzard G, Konstantakopoulou E, Garway-Heath D, et al. Selective laser trabeculoplasty versus eye drops for first-line treatment of ocular hypertension and glaucoma (LiGHT): a multicentre randomised controlled trial. Lancet 2019; 393(10180):1505–16.

47. Azuara-Blanco A, Burr J, Ramsay C, et al. Effectiveness of early lens extraction for the treatment of primary angle-closure glaucoma (EAGLE): a randomised controlled trial. Lancet 2016;388(10052):1389–97.

48. Bain WE. The fellow eye in acute closed-angle glaucoma. Br J Ophthalmol 1957; 41(4):193–9.

49. Guedes GB, Karan A, Mayer HR, et al. Evaluation of adverse events in self-reported sulfa-allergic patients using topical carbonic anhydrase inhibitors. J Ocul Pharmacol Ther 2013;29(5):456–61.

50. Tanna AP, Rademaker AW, Stewart WC, et al. Meta-analysis of the efficacy and safety of alpha2-adrenergic agonists, beta-adrenergic antagonists, and topical carbonic anhydrase inhibitors with prostaglandin analogs. Arch Ophthalmol 2010;128(7):825–33.

51. Flach AJ. The importance of eyelid closure and nasolacrimal occlusion following the ocular instillation of topical glaucoma medications, and the need for the universal inclusion of one of these techniques in all patient treatments and clinical studies. Trans Am Ophthalmol Soc 2008;106:138–48.

52. Alvarado JA, Shifera AS. Progress towards understanding the functioning of the trabecular meshwork based on lessons from studies of laser trabeculoplasty. Br J Ophthalmol 2010;94(11):1417–8.

53. Napier ML, Azuara-Blanco A. Changing patterns in treatment of angle closure glaucoma. Curr Opin Ophthalmol 2018;29(2).

54. Vinod K, Gedde SJ. Safety profile of minimally invasive glaucoma surgery. Curr Opin Ophthalmol 2021;32(2):160–8. https://doi.org/10.1097/ICU.0000000000000731. PMID: 33315726.

55. Lavia C, Dallorto L, Maule M, et al. Minimally-invasive glaucoma surgeries (MIGS) for open angle glaucoma: A systematic review and meta-analysis. PLoS One 2017;12(8):e0183142.
56. Gedde SJ, Scott IU, Tabandeh H, et al. Late endophthalmitis associated with glaucoma drainage implants. Ophthalmology 2001;108(7):1323–7.
57. Kangas TA, Greenfield DS, Flynn HW Jr, et al. Delayed-onset endophthalmitis associated with conjunctival filtering blebs. Ophthalmology 1997;104(5): 746–52.

# Neuro-Ophthalmology for Internists

Neena R. Cherayil, MD[a,b,*], Madhura A. Tamhankar, MD[c]

## KEYWORDS

- Vision loss • Double vision • Unequal pupils • Neuro-ophthalmology

## KEY POINTS

- Testing visual fields to confrontation in each eye separately can localize vision loss to the eye, optic nerve, chiasm, or postchiasmal optic pathways.
- The clinical approach to examining those with unequal size pupils should first focus on identifying which pupil is abnormal by observing the asymmetry of pupil size in ambient and dim-lighting conditions.
- Monocular double vision that persists even when 1 eye is occluded is almost always a result of ophthalmic disease and should be evaluated by an ophthalmologist nonurgently.
- Binocular double vision that resolves with occlusion of either eye implies a misalignment of visual axes and can result from a variety of causes, including ocular motor nerve palsy, skew deviation, internuclear ophthalmoplegia, myasthenia gravis, thyroid eye disease, and strabismus.

 Video content accompanies this article at http://www.medical.theclinics.com.

## NEURO-OPHTHALMIC CAUSES OF ACUTE VISION LOSS
### Clinics Care Points

- Testing visual fields to confrontation in each eye separately can localize vision loss to the eye, optic nerve, chiasm, or postchiasmal pathways.
- Giant cell arteritis can cause acute monocular vision loss as a result of arteritic ischemic optic neuropathy in adults older than the age of 55 years. Prompt treatment with high-dose intravenous steroids is required to prevent further vision loss and morbidity.
- Nonarteritic ischemic optic neuropathy presents with acute altitudinal monocular vision loss often noted on waking in adults older than the age of 50 years with

[a] Department of Neurology, Northwestern University, 259 E. Erie St, Ste 1520, Chicago, IL 60611, USA; [b] Department of Ophthalmology, Northwestern University, Chicago, IL, USA; [c] Department of Ophthalmology, University of Pennsylvania, 51 N 39th St, Philadelphia, PA 19104, USA
* Corresponding author.
E-mail address: neena.cherayil@gmail.com

Med Clin N Am 105 (2021) 511–529
https://doi.org/10.1016/j.mcna.2021.01.005
0025-7125/21/© 2021 Elsevier Inc. All rights reserved.

vascular risk factors, including obstructive sleep apnea and use of drugs for erectile dysfunction.

- Optic neuritis typically presents in younger women (aged 20–40 years) with vision loss, decrease in color vision, and pain with eye movements evolving over hours to days. Patients with optic neuritis should be referred for MRI brain imaging and neurology to stratify risk for developing demyelinating disease.
- Vision loss associated with migraine is exceedingly common but can be difficult to distinguish from other ocular processes. Migraine aura is typified by mixed positive and negative phenomena, such as an area of vision loss surrounded by shimmering edges (scintillating scotoma) that evolves over 15 to 30 minutes.

## BACKGROUND

Patients with sudden monocular vision loss have a disorder of the eye, retina, or optic nerve anywhere along its course.[1] Patients with neuro-ophthalmic causes of vision loss tend to be more definitive in their description of vision loss with regard to onset, duration, and semiology. Patients with ophthalmic causes of vision loss may describe long-standing, vague visual blurring, haziness, distortion, fogging, or monocular diplopia. Monocular amaurosis or "fleeting blindness," often described as a shade or veil coming over one's vision, is highly suggestive of a retinal-vascular event because of a temporary interruption of retinal circulation, including central or branch retinal artery occlusion.[2,3] These causes are described further in the retina article of this issue. This section focuses on common presentations of common neuro-ophthalmic disorders causing vision loss.

## APPROACH TO ACUTE VISION LOSS

Neuro-ophthalmic processes involving a visual field defect in both eyes can localize to the bilateral optic nerves, optic chiasm, or the optic pathways within the brain. Patients with post–chiasmal intracranial lesions will have homonymous vision loss, that is, a visual field defect on the same side in each eye.[1] Often these patients may only notice a nasal field defect and may only complain of vision loss in the eye with temporal field loss. Testing visual fields to confrontation in each eye separately is thus of crucial importance. Homonymous field loss can be caused by mass lesion, cerebral ischemia or hypoperfusion, migraine, or seizure. Patients with mass, stroke, and seizure will often have a history of associated focal neurologic deficits, although isolated homonymous visual field defects can be seen with occipital lobe lesions without accompanying neurologic features.

### Giant cell arteritis

Temporal arteritis or giant cell arteritis (GCA) is a neuro-ophthalmic emergency and is one of the most feared causes of acute vision loss, as it can rapidly progress to blindness and other vasculitic complications if not diagnosed and treated early. GCA is the most common systemic vasculitis in people older than 50 years of age.[4] Prevalence of GCA increases with age, and most affected patients are older than 70 years.[5,6] Women are affected at rates 2 to 3 times higher than that of men, similar to other autoimmune diseases.[7] GCA causes ischemia of target tissues via inflammatory narrowing or occlusion of mid- to large-sized vessels[7,8] and preferentially affects the extradural and superficial vessels, including the temporal, vertebral, ophthalmic, and posterior ciliary arteries,[8,9] leading to a high frequency of visual complications. GCA can present with exclusively systemic involvement, exclusively ophthalmic involvement, or both.

Isolated ophthalmic presentation is known as occult GCA and is reported to account for 20% to 38% of GCA with ophthalmic involvement.[8,10]

Affected individuals commonly experience sudden transient or permanent vision loss from optic nerve, retinal, or, more rarely, intracranial ischemia. Vision loss in GCA is acute and severe and occasionally accompanied by pain. Bilateral vision loss can occur in up to 62% of patients, and many patients with GCA report preceding episodes of blurring or darkening of their vision before the permanent event.[2,3,8] Arteritic anterior ischemic optic neuropathy (AAION), presenting with pallid swelling of the optic nerve head owing to ischemia (**Fig. 1**), is responsible for most vision loss in GCA.[2,8,10,11] Untreated patients can go on to develop second eye involvement rapidly, often in a matter of days to weeks.[2,11,12] Double vision (with or without vision loss) as a result of ischemia of the extraocular muscles or ocular motor cranial nerves is a rarer presenting symptom of GCA reported in up to 15% of patients.[5,11,13]

A careful history with attention to the presence of constitutional symptoms (fever, malaise, weight loss), headache, scalp tenderness, head/temple pain, jaw claudication with chewing or talking, and proximal myalgias must be performed. Palpation of the temporal arteries may reveal point tenderness, palpable cords, or absent pulses.[2] In older patients presenting with transient vision loss, GCA is on the differential diagnosis, and practitioners should inquire about the presence of constitutional symptoms.

Erythrocyte sedimentation rate (ESR) and C-reactive protein (CRP) are acute phase reactants elevated in GCA and must be sent for all patients with suspicious ophthalmic or systemic symptoms even if transient. The combination of both tests is 97% specific for GCA.[14,15] Normocytic anemia and thrombocytosis may also be seen.[15-17] It is rare for a patient with GCA, including occult GCA, to have both normal ESR/CRP and absence of systemic symptoms.[8,18,19] Prompt high-dose corticosteroid treatment prevents further vision loss and occasionally provides symptomatic relief.[8,20] When in doubt and GCA is being considered, the authors recommend treating patients with corticosteroids while the diagnosis is pursued. Duplex ultrasound of the superficial temporal artery may support a diagnosis of GCA with visualization of arterial stenosis, occlusion, or vessel wall edema, although overall sensitivity is low.[21,22]

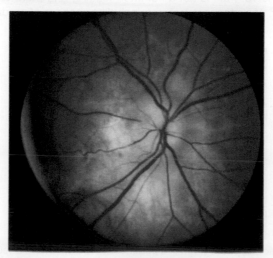

**Fig. 1.** Right eye fundus photograph in a patient with GCA. Notice the pallid optic nerve swelling indicating arteritic anterior ischemic optic neuropathy.

High-resolution MRI with contrast can also assess temporal artery mural thickness and patency with submillimeter resolution.[23] Temporal artery biopsy (TAB) continues to be the gold standard for the diagnosis of GCA. Long-segment (>3 cm) TAB is a low-risk diagnostic procedure and will show necrotic inflammation in the arterial media with multinucleated giant cells or epithelioid macrophages.[19,24,25] Pathologic evidence of GCA can be seen even after a week of high-dose steroid treatment, so treatment should not be withheld while awaiting biopsy.[19,24] TAB can be negative in many clinically suspected cases as a result of skip lesions. Contralateral biopsy is recommended in these cases to establish diagnosis.

The treatment of GCA involves high-dose steroids followed by prolonged taper. Additional immunosuppression may be required if there is a relapse of symptoms.[20] Recent studies on the use of tocilizumab, a monoclonal antibody blocking the interleukin 6 receptor, have been promising. Patients with visual symptoms should be managed long term by both the rheumatologist and the ophthalmologist working in conjunction.

### Nonarteritic anterior ischemic optic neuropathy

Nonarteritic anterior ischemic optic neuropathy (NAION) is the most common cause of acute unilateral vision loss in adults older than the age of 50 years, causes sectoral optic nerve head swelling often accompanied by disc hemorrhage (**Fig. 2**), and typically occurs in patients with vascular risk factors.[24,26–28] NAION occurs as a result of microvascular ischemia to the optic nerve head, which is supplied radially by branches of the posterior ciliary arteries and is a potential watershed area.[24] A cupless optic nerve, also known as a "disc at risk," is the strongest risk factor for the development of NAION and is thought to cause a "compartment syndrome" at the time of ischemia.[24,27] Nocturnal hypotension, obstructive sleep apnea, and the use of erectile dysfunction drugs may be distinct risk factors, as they predispose to relative hypoperfusion of the optic nerve head in the already vulnerable patient.[29–33]

Patients with NAION will typically present with acute monocular vision loss, maximal at onset and often noted on waking.[34] Vision loss is confined to 1 eye and is often altitudinal (**Fig. 3**), that is, respecting the horizontal meridian as a result of sectoral infarction of the optic nerve. Pain is not a common feature, and there are no associated neurologic, ocular, or systemic symptoms, including absence of prodromal symptoms

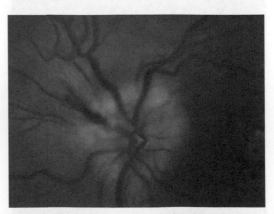

**Fig. 2.** Left eye optic disc photograph in a patient with NAION. There is sectoral superior optic nerve swelling with associated flame-shaped hemorrhage superonasally characteristic of NAION.

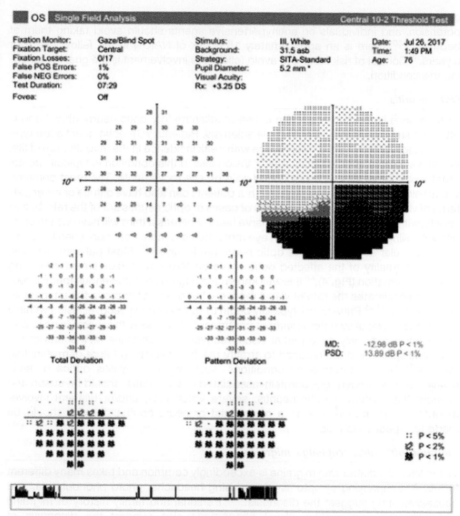

**Fig. 3.** Left eye Humphrey visual field testing for the patient represented in **Fig. 2**. There is inferior altitudinal visual field loss in respect to the horizontal. MD, mean deviation; NEG, negative; POS, positive; PSD, pattern standard deviation; SITA, Swedish Interactive Threshold Algorithm.

for GCA.[27] Vision loss is not as severe as in patients presenting with AAION, with nearly half of patients presenting with vision better than 20/70 at initial presentation, although up to one-third can have vision worse than 20/200.[24,28] Patients with NAION can have some spontaneous improvement or progression of vision loss in the first 4 weeks after onset.

Given the overlap in presentation of GCA causing AAION, evaluation of patients with NAION should include review of constitutional symptoms associated with GCA and consideration of serum ESR/CRP.[24]

Despite several trials investigating a variety of interventions from aspirin to optic nerve decompression, there is currently no effective treatment for NAION.[30] Regardless, affected individuals should be evaluated for and counseled on control of modifiable risk factors, such as diabetes mellitus, hypertension, hyperlipidemia, smoking cessation, and obstructive sleep apnea. Care should be taken to avoid nocturnal hypotension, and individuals on antihypertensive agents should avoid taking them at bedtime.[29,30] There is an approximately 15% risk of NAION in the fellow eye over 5 years.[35] Control of risk factors to avoid fellow eye involvement is the goal in managing this condition.

### Optic neuritis

Optic neuritis is the most common cause of inflammatory optic neuropathy[24] and is often the first manifestation of multiple sclerosis. Patients with optic neuritis are typically young women of child-bearing age with peak incidence in the third decade of life. Women are more affected than men.[36] Vision loss in this condition is typically acute, progressing over days with associated pain on eye movements. The most common visual field defect is a central scotoma, but patients can also have diffuse or other patterns of visual field loss.[37,38] Two-thirds of cases of optic neuritis are of the retrobulbar variety, with normal-appearing optic nerve head, whereas a third will have visible optic nerve swelling. Eye pain or pain with eye movements is more common when longer or intracanalicular segments of the optic nerve are involved.[39] Most patients will have some abnormality of the affected optic nerve on MRI with enhancement indicating active inflammation (**Fig. 4**).[40] It is well known that high-dose intravenous methylprednisolone accelerates the rate of visual recovery but does not improve the ultimate visual outcome.[41,42] Patients will typically begin to spontaneously recover vision within a month after onset of symptoms without treatment.[42,43] Those with severe vision loss at presentation may only have partial visual recovery.[42,43] Baseline MRI scans of the brain and spinal cord are required to stratify risk for developing future demyelinating disease.[24] Other demyelinating conditions, such as neuromyelitis optica or anti–myelin-oligodendrocyte-glycoprotein–associated optic neuritis, should be suspected in those with recurrent optic neuritis, severe vision loss, and/or bilateral involvement.[24,44–46] Prompt referral to a neurologist or neuro-ophthalmologist should be made to expedite work up.

### Migraine with aura, acephalgic migraine

Vision loss associated with migraine is exceedingly common and takes many different forms. Accompanying symptoms of throbbing headache, photo phonophobia, and nausea/vomiting suggest the diagnosis.[2,47] Personal and family history of migraine and accompanying positive visual phenomena also support the diagnosis of migrainous visual loss. Migrainous visual symptoms can be in 1 eye or both eyes and frequently manifest as scintillating scotoma, hemianopia, or monocular visual loss. The best example of combined negative and positive visual phenomena in

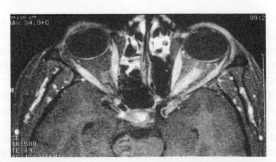

**Fig. 4.** Postcontrast T1-weighted axial MRI of the orbits revealing diffuse contrast enhancement of the left optic nerve.

migraine is an enlarging scintillating scotoma described as an area of blurry, wavy, or absent vision surrounded by shimmering colors.[2] Some migraine patients may develop a true hemianopia in the aura phase without positive visual phenomena often building up over several minutes and then resolving over 15 to 30 minutes but may only notice it in 1 eye. Some patients may complain of monocular scotoma or complete loss of vision in 1 eye for seconds or minutes. Patients generally do not describe classical amaurosis with "a shade coming down" over their vision as occurs with embolic retinal artery occlusion.[48,49]

Nonembolic monocular vision loss is more likely to present with positive visual symptoms in contrast to embolic vision loss, which is characterized by a blackout of vision.[2,49] Purely negative phenomena, although they can occur in migraine aura, are unusual. The exact pathophysiology of vision changes in migraine is not known, but likely mechanisms include vasospasm and nonischemic cortical spreading depression.[50,51]

In classic migraine with aura, a typical migraine headache with unilateral hemicranial throbbing, photo phonophobia, and nausea with emesis follows visual disturbance. Older patients, many with a history of migraines as younger adults, can develop migrainous visual aura without headache, so-called acephalgic migraine. Often, these events can be difficult to distinguish from an ischemic embolic event, such as branch retinal artery occlusion. When positive visual phenomena and gradual build-up of aura symptoms occur over 15 to 30 minutes, migraine is more readily differentiated from an occipital lobe transient ischemic attack or seizure.[2] Rarely, occipital lobe lesions, such as meningioma or arteriovenous malformations, can mimic migraine. Meningioma or arteriovenous malformations should be suspected and ruled out with MRI in any patients with atypical symptoms or with a crescendo of increased frequency or intensity of vision loss episodes.

## UNEQUAL PUPILS
### Clinics Care Points

- The clinical approach to unequally sized pupils should first focus on identifying which pupil is abnormal by observing the asymmetry of pupil size in ambient and dim-lighting conditions.
- An abnormally constricted pupil is often the result of sympathetic pathway disruption (Horner syndrome) and is accompanied by mild upper- and lower-lid ptosis and anhidrosis. Patients presenting with new Horner syndrome should be urgently evaluated with contrast MRI of the brain, vessel imaging of the head and neck, and chest imaging to rule out compressive mass lesion or carotid dissection.
- Central first- and second-order Horner lesions are accompanied by adjacent neurologic signs.
- An abnormally dilated pupil can result from parasympathetic pathway interruption, most concerningly, a third nerve palsy, damage to iris sphincter muscle, Adie tonic pupil, or pharmacologic effect.

## APPROACH TO HISTORY AND EXAMINATION OF PATIENT WITH UNEQUAL PUPILS

Anisocoria or unequal pupils can be due to a variety of harmless or life-threatening causes and is easily examined in a general practice setting. The history should focus on when pupillary asymmetry was noted, associated neck or head pain, history of head, neck, or ocular trauma, and prior history of ocular surgery. Review of prior photographs, including driver's license, is useful to determine if anisocoria is long-standing. Red flag symptoms include presence of eye/head/neck pain and associated neurologic symptoms, such as diplopia, ptosis, ataxia, or focal weakness and numbness. In appropriate cases, patients should additionally be queried regarding carotid dissection risk factors, including head and neck trauma, whiplash, or torsional neck injury, such as chiropractic adjustment, or prolonged neck extension. History of cancer, unintentional weight loss, and other constitutional symptoms might increase suspicion for compressive primary or secondary mass.

A careful review of a patient's medication list and potential exposures is essential in patients presenting with anisocoria, as pharmacologic exposure is a common benign cause of abnormal pupillary dilation (mydriasis) or constriction (miosis), as discussed later. Physicians should specifically ask about use of nasal sprays, topical medicinal patches or wipes, inhalers, nebulizers, supplements as well as exposures to pesticides or plants with adrenergic or cholinergic properties.

The clinical approach to examining anisocoria should first focus on identifying which pupil is abnormal by observing the asymmetry of pupil size in bright- and dim-lighting conditions. A greater difference between size of pupils in bright light indicates that the larger pupil is unable to constrict appropriately to light, implying parasympathetic dysfunction. Conversely, a greater degree of anisocoria in darker conditions indicates the smaller pupil is abnormal with sympathetic dysfunction impeding appropriate pupil dilation in the absence of light.

## PHYSIOLOGIC ANISOCORIA

Physiologic anisocoria is a common benign cause of asymmetric pupils occurring in up to 1 in 5 of the American population according to some studies.[52] Review of old photographs is helpful for establishing the long-standing nature of asymmetric pupils. Patients with physiologic anisocoria should have normal extraocular motility, lid position and function, and pupillary reactivity with a degree of anisocoria remaining similar in bright and dim light.

## ANISOCORIA DUE TO ABNORMALLY CONSTRICTED PUPIL
### Horner syndrome

- A 3-neuron sympathetic arc is responsible for catecholaminergic pupillary dilation. The first-order neuron in the hypothalamus descends through the brainstem to synapse in the lower-cervical/upper-thoracic spinal cord. The second-order neuron exits the sympathetic chain and traverses the upper chest and neck to reach the third-order neuron in the cervical ganglion at the bifurcation of the common carotid artery. The third-order neuron adheres to the internal carotid artery in the neck and intracranially through the cavernous sinus before finally coursing forward and terminating in the orbit. Interruption anywhere along this system is responsible for the classic triad of "ptosis, miosis, and anhidrosis" known as Horner syndrome.[53]
- Horner syndrome can result from compression, infarction, or inflammation or demyelination anywhere along the protracted 3-neuron course. Central first- and second-order Horner syndrome is accompanied by neurologic "neighborhood signs." A lateral medullary brainstem stroke, for example, would present acutely with Horner syndrome because of involvement of descending first-order sympathetic tract with associated hemi-facial and hemi-body sensory dysfunction, dysphagia, dysarthria, and asymmetric tongue protrusion or vertigo and ataxia with cerebellar involvement. The second-order neuron can be compressed as it travels through the chest and neck, most classically by apical

lung mass (Pancoast tumor). Internal carotid artery dissection can cause third-order Horner syndrome. Associated pain is a red flag sign and can accompany carotid dissection, cavernous sinus, or orbital lesion.[53,54]

- Patients with miosis owing to Horner syndrome will have anisocoria more prominent in the dark and may demonstrate pupillary "dilation lag" whereby the abnormal pupil takes 5 to 10 seconds to enlarge and "catch up" to the contralateral eye when lights are dim.[53]
- The ptosis of Horner syndrome is due to sympathetic denervation of the superior and inferior tarsal muscles (Muller muscle), which causes lowering of the upper lid and elevation of the lower lid (so-called inverse ptosis). As a result, the affected eye may appear smaller because of a narrower palpebral fissure (**Fig. 5**). The ptosis of Horner syndrome is mild and never complete; moderate to severe ptosis in a patient with suspected Horner should prompt consideration of alternative causes of eyelid drooping.[53]
- Facial anhidrosis or absence of sweating results from proximal first- and second-order sympathetic nerve dysfunction, as the sudomotor fibers of this pathway synapse at the cervical ganglion in the neck and travel with the external carotid artery to the face rather than with the third-order neuron along the internal carotid artery. Patients may note decreased sweating or hyperemia of the ipsilateral face with exertion relative to the contralateral side (**Fig. 6**).[53]
- Patients with congenital or infantile Horner syndrome may have asymmetric iris color (heterochromia, lighter on the affected side), as early sympathetic tone is required for melanocyte pigmentation in the iris stroma.[55,56]
- Adult patients with new or acute Horner syndrome merit urgent evaluation with contrast MRI of the brain, contrast vessel imaging of the head and neck down to the level of T2 to include the subclavian artery and lung apices. More than one-third of patients with confirmed Horner syndrome will be idiopathic with unremarkable imaging.[54,57,58]

## Other causes of abnormally constricted pupil

- In the long term, an Adie tonic pupil, as discussed in the next section, results in an abnormally constricted pupil.[53]
- Pharmacologic agents that could potentially cause asymmetric pupillary constriction include topical opiates (fentanyl patch), clonidine patch, pilocarpine eye drops, and organophosphate insecticides but are a much less noted cause of pharmacologic anisocoria than pharmacologic dilation.

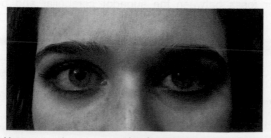

**Fig. 5.** A left-sided Horner syndrome as result of cervical spine arteriovenous malformation rupture. Note smaller pupil on the left with accompanying upper-lid ptosis and lower-lid "inverse ptosis."

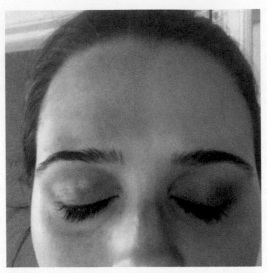

**Fig. 6.** Lack of hyperemia with exercise on the affected side in the patient from **Fig. 5** with left-sided second-order Horner syndrome.

## ANISOCORIA DUE TO ABNORMALLY DILATED PUPIL

Efferent reflex pupil constriction to light and near is mediated by the parasympathetic pupillomotor fibers, which travel with cranial nerve 3 and synapse in the ciliary ganglion within the orbit before traveling to the pupillary sphincter. An abnormally dilated pupil can thus be a result of direct iris trauma or inflammation, ciliary ganglion lesion, or peripheral or central cranial nerve 3 involvement.[53]

### Third nerve palsy

- The most concerning and potentially life-threatening cause for a dilated pupil is a third nerve palsy. Signs and symptoms of third nerve palsy include diplopia as result of impaired extraocular movements, significant upper-lid ptosis, and dilated pupil greater than 5 mm with sluggish reactivity (**Fig. 7**). Pupil-involving third nerve palsies are often compressive given the distribution of the pupillomotor fibers on the external dorsomedial surface of the third cranial nerve.[53,59]
- Cranial nerve 3 is particularly susceptible to compression by aneurysm, as it exits the posterior fossa between the superior cerebellar and posterior cerebral

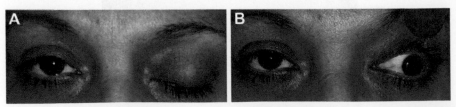

**Fig. 7.** (*A*) Complete ptosis in a patient with a left third nerve palsy from compressive posterior communicating artery aneurysm. (*B*) Note left eye is deviated "down and out" when the eyelid is elevated with dilated pupil.

arteries. Isolated pupillary dilation from third nerve palsy is rare, but evolving compressive lesions, especially enlarging aneurysm, can present with pupil dilation before development of extraocular dysmotility or ptosis.[60] Most cases of aneurysmal compression are painful, although slow-growing aneurysms can present similarly to slow-growing tumors like meningioma.

- Patients with third nerve palsy from evolving brainstem herniation will have altered mental status (often obtundation) and headaches or nausea/vomiting from increased intracranial pressure. They develop an acutely dilated and nonreactive pupil from compression of the ipsilateral third nerve from the uncus of the temporal lobe as it herniates inferiorly through the tentorium cerebelli.[53] These patients are not encountered in the routine outpatient setting.

- Midbrain infarction or hemorrhage affecting third nerve nucleus will have signs and symptoms of third nerve palsy associated with other focal neurologic symptoms, including contralateral weakness, hemiataxia or choreoathetosis, or parkinsonism or rubral tremor.[61]

### Adie tonic pupil

- A monocular dilated pupil can occasionally be a result of Adie tonic pupil. In this idiopathic, benign condition that typically affects young women, patients develop irregularly shaped dilated pupil with slow constriction to light and sluggish redilation. Constriction of the pupil to near will be relatively preserved because of the increased 30:1 ratio of parasympathetic fibers mediating the near reflex.[53]

- The syndrome is definitively diagnosed by slit-lamp examination for sectoral hypokinesis and vermiform writhing movements of the iris and dilute pilocarpine testing, which can be performed in an ophthalmology or neuro-ophthalmology office. Adie tonic pupil is thought to result from idiopathic damage to the ciliary ganglion and is monocular in 80% of cases. Occasionally, tonic dilated pupils can be a result of GCA,[62] orbital inflammation or neoplasm,[63,64] sarcoidosis,[65] autonomic disorder,[66] or Guillain-Barre syndrome.[67] When associated with areflexia, it is termed Holmes-Adie syndrome.

### Pharmacologically dilated pupil

- Accidental ocular exposure to sympathomimetic drugs (phenylephrine, cocaine, nasal vasoconstrictors) or anticholinergic medications (ipratropium, scopolamine, glycopyrrolate drops/wipes, tropicamide, Datura or Solanum plant species) is common.[68-71] A review of the patient's medication list and possible exposures is essential, but the offending agent sometimes cannot be identified. The pupil is typically maximally dilated and fixed. Pharmacologic dilation should resolve with removal of culprit medication. Two-step pilocarpine drop testing in the ophthalmologist's office is diagnostic.[71,72] Practitioners should closely examine eyelid function and extraocular motility to rule out third nerve palsy.

## NEW-ONSET DOUBLE VISION
### Clinics Care Points

- Monocular double vision that persists even when 1 eye is occluded is almost always a result of ophthalmic disease and should be evaluated by an ophthalmologist nonurgently.

- Patients presenting with isolated ocular motor nerve palsy (third, fourth, or sixth nerve) should also undergo MRI brain with and without contrast, regardless of age. In addition, all patients with new third nerve palsy should be urgently evaluated with intracranial vascular imaging to rule out compressive aneurysm.

- Expedited contrast-enhanced MRI should be included in the diagnostic work up in patients who present with acute onset of binocular diplopia with or without extraocular motility deficit to rule out brainstem ischemia, inflammation, or intracranial compressive lesions causing internuclear ophthalmoplegia or skew deviation.
- Myasthenia gravis can mimic any pattern of ocular misalignment and is often accompanied by fatigable ptosis. Pupils are not affected in this condition.

## BACKGROUND

Double vision is a common presenting complaint in both ambulatory and inpatient settings and is frequently encountered in neurology and ophthalmology practices.[73–75] Those presenting with new-onset diplopia require immediate diagnostic evaluation and management to prevent morbidity and mortality.

Initial evaluation of a patient presenting with double vision is to determine whether the double image disappears with occlusion of 1 eye. Patients who have persistence of double images even when 1 eye is occluded have monocular double vision, which is rarely caused by neurologic disease and is often described as "ghost images" or shadows.[76] It is important to elucidate if the patient has resolution with occlusion of *either* eye, as patients who have single-eye monocular diplopia will report resolution of double vision with closure of the affected eye. Monocular double vision can be ascribed to benign causes, such as uncorrected refractive error, corneal defects, including ocular surface disease, such as dry eye, ocular media opacity, such as cataract, or macular disease.[77,78] Patients with isolated monocular diplopia should be reassured and nonurgently referred to an optometrist or ophthalmologist for further evaluation.

Patients who report resolution of double vision with occlusion of either eye have binocular diplopia, which occurs as a result of ocular misalignment. Of note, there are patients who can have cooccurrence of monocular and binocular diplopia. These patients should be referred to an ophthalmologist or neuro-ophthalmologist for stepwise and comprehensive evaluation of their complaint.

## HISTORY IN THE PATIENT WITH DOUBLE VISION

Patients presenting with new-onset diplopia should be evaluated urgently. Providers can arrive at a neuroanatomical localization of a patient's diplopia by history alone, querying if the double images are horizontally, vertically, or obliquely displaced or tilted, whether distance between images becomes more or less prominent in a particular direction of gaze or head tilt, and whether images are further apart at distance or near.[76] Semiology of symptoms, including duration and progression, whether symptoms are intermittent, constant, or task-specific, and whether there is fatigability, is also important in differential diagnosis of diplopia; for instance, variable diplopia that worsens with exertion and resolves with rest should increase the index of suspicion for myasthenia gravis.[76,79]

In many patients, diplopia may be an isolated finding, but the examining physician must also determine if there is a history of other neurologic signs or symptoms, such as headache, eye pain, vision loss, ptosis, anisocoria, or weakness and numbness of the face or extremities and ataxia that might implicate a worrisome central cause of symptoms.[79] A history of vasculopathic risk factors, such as diabetes mellitus, hypertension, hyperlipidemia, coronary/peripheral artery disease, and smoking history, should be sought, as these conditions increase the risk of microvascular ischemic cranial neuropathies. In patients older than 50 years, systemic symptoms of GCA, such as jaw claudication, lingual ulcers, scalp/temporal tenderness, weight loss, and other constitutional symptoms, should also be surveyed, as diplopia is rarely the presenting sign of this vision-threatening condition and is reported to occur in 2% to 15% of patients with GCA.[13,76]

Other relevant causes of diplopia that should be surveyed include past history of strabismus with prior eye muscle surgery, head or orbital trauma, prior orbital disease, signs and symptoms of thyroid dysfunction, cancer, or neurologic disease, and history of prior neurosurgical intervention.

### Isolated ocular motor cranial nerve palsies

A 2014 study found that over half of patients with new diplopia presented isolated third, fourth, or sixth cranial nerve palsy.[79] The diagnosis of ocular motor cranial nerve palsies can be made on examination of extraocular movements and alignment. Patients with a third nerve palsy present with ptosis and eye deviating "down and out" with variable presence of adduction, elevation, and/or depression deficits (Video 1). The pupil may be involved with abnormal dilation as mentioned in the anisocoria subsection. Patients with a fourth nerve palsy present with vertical or oblique diplopia, often with subtle tilting of double image, that worsens in contralateral gaze and ipsilateral head tilt. Extraocular movements often appear full in patients with fourth nerve palsy. Sixth nerve palsy is characterized by the presence of binocular horizontal diplopia with an abduction deficit on the involved side (Video 2) and eye deviating inwards that increases on lateral gaze to the side of the palsy.[76]

### Diagnosis and treatment of isolated ocular motor cranial nerve palsy

The causes of acute-onset isolated ocular motor cranial neuropathies include ischemia, compression, inflammation, infiltration, trauma, and neuromuscular junction disorders. Certain causes are more commonly associated with specific ocular motor cranial nerves.[80] In those who present with acute third nerve palsy, pupil involvement is critical to ascertain. In pupil-involving third nerve palsies, compressive lesions, particularly posterior communicating artery aneurysms, are an important consideration, as mentioned in the anisocoria subsection. Such patients must be emergently referred to the emergency room (ER) to rule out intracranial aneurysm. Congenital dysgenesis of the trochlear nerve/superior oblique complex is the most common cause of fourth nerve palsy, although it can present later in life in adults as insidious onset of vertical diplopia. The fourth cranial nerve is also commonly involved in closed head trauma because of its smaller size and circuitous course from dorsal midbrain to orbit. Sixth nerve palsies can result from raised intracranial pressure, compressive skull base lesions, or head trauma.

In adults older than age 50 years, isolated fourth, sixth, and pupil-sparing third cranial neuropathies frequently occur from presumed microvascular ischemia in the setting of atherosclerotic risk factors.[80–82] The sixth cranial nerve is the most commonly involved.81 These ischemic cranial neuropathies have excellent prognosis for spontaneous recovery, typically with full resolution over the course of 3 to 6 months.[76,81]

Multiple older retrospective studies have found variable incidence between 1.1% and 13.5% of causes other than microvascular ischemia in patients presenting with acute isolated ocular motor palsy. The sole multicenter prospective study on neuroimaging in these patients found that 16.5% of patients had nonmicrovascular causes for their symptoms, including pituitary apoplexy, mass lesions, brainstem infarction whereby early intervention can prevent considerable morbidity and mortality.[82] The investigators found that although the presence of vasculopathic risk factors was a significant predictor for presumed microvascular cause, 61% of patients who harbored other causes of isolated ocular motor cranial neuropathy also harbored at least 1 vascular risk factor. The investigators concluded that contrast-enhanced brain MRI plays an important role in evaluation of patients with acute isolated ocular motor mononeuropathies even in older adults. Cost-effectiveness of early MRI compared favorably with accepted practices in imaging patients with headaches and nonfocal neurologic examinations.[81,82]

## Skew Deviation

A skew deviation refers to an acquired vertical misalignment of the eyes that occurs as a result of posterior fossa lesions that disrupt the utricular-vestibular-ocular pathways, which includes the medial longitudinal fasciculus (MLF), in the brainstem.[76,83,84] This pathway governs the vertical and rotational position of the eye in response to body tilt and is often affected by acute brainstem stroke. Skew deviation may present with acute vertical diplopia with or without ataxia, vertigo, and weakness. In such patients, suspicion of brainstem stroke is high, and these patients should be referred to the nearest ER for stroke evaluation.[83]

## Internuclear Ophthalmoplegia

Disruption of the MLF in the pons or midbrain results in internuclear ophthalmoplegia (INO), which is characterized by slowed adduction in 1 eye and contralateral abducting nystagmus.[85] Convergence is typically preserved in pontine lesions because cranial nerve 3 is unaffected (Video 3). Patients can present with diplopia worse in contralateral gaze and may have oblique diplopia if there is a concomitant skew deviation. Patients with subtle adduction weakness may have no symptoms or only complain of blurred vision with eccentric or quick shifts in horizontal gaze.[76] Bilateral lesions of the MLF often produce additional eye findings, including impaired vertical pursuit and upbeat nystagmus in both eyes in upgaze. One should carefully search for other orbital signs, because isolated medial rectus lesions may occur from local conditions, such as extraocular muscle entrapment, typically when there is eye trauma. Third nerve palsy should be considered, and ptosis, mydriasis, and vertical eye movement impairment should be carefully excluded. Unilateral INO in an older patient usually results from brainstem stroke,[86] whereas unilateral or bilateral INO in a young patient typically signifies a demyelinating process, such as multiple sclerosis. In both causes, the prognosis for spontaneous improvement over weeks is excellent.[87]

## Myasthenia Gravis

Ptosis and extraocular dysmotility are seen in most patients with myasthenia gravis, an autoimmune disease caused by circulating antibodies that block effective communication between acetylcholine and post–synaptic receptors in the neuromuscular junction.[88] About half of patients present with ptosis or extraocular motility defects only, and, of this group, half will remain ocular, whereas others go on to develop generalized weakness, including prominent proximal greater than distal muscle weakness and bulbar weakness presenting as dysphagia, dysarthria, hypophonia, or respiratory insufficiency.[76,89] The onset of ptosis and diplopia usually progresses in a subacute manner over weeks. Ocular myasthenia gravis can affect any extraocular muscle, and the motility and alignment pattern may mimic any pupil-sparing cause of diplopia, including third, fourth, or sixth cranial neuropathy, INO, skew deviation, or gaze palsy. Anti-acetylcholine-receptor antibody levels are abnormal in half of patients with isolated ocular myasthenia, and electromyography with repetitive nerve stimulation and single-fiber studies are important adjunct tests. Early referral to neuromuscular or neuro-ophthalmology specialist is ideal.

## DISCLOSURE

The authors have no relevant disclosures.

## SUPPLEMENTARY DATA

Supplementary data related to this article can be found online at https://doi.org/10.1016/j.mcna.2021.01.005.

## REFERENCES

1. Liu GT, Volpe NJ, Galetta SL. Visual loss: overview, visual field testing, and topical diagnosis. In: Liu, Volpe, and Galetta's neuro-ophthalmology. 3rd ed. ; 2019:39-52. Available at: https://www-clinicalkey-com.ezproxy.galter.northwestern.edu/#!/content/book/3-s2.0-B9780323340441000031. Accessed October 21, 2020.
2. Tamhankar MA. Transient visual loss or blurring. In: Liu, Volpe, and Galetta's neuro-ophthalmology. 3rd ed. ; 2019:365-377. Available at: https://www-clinicalkey-com.ezproxy.galter.northwestern.edu/#!/content/book/3-s2.0-B9780323340441000109. Accessed September 19, 2020.
3. Hayreh SS, Zimmerman MB. Amaurosis fugax in ocular vascular occlusive disorders: prevalence and pathogeneses. Retina 2014;34(1):115–22.
4. Garrity ST, Pistilli M, Vaphiades MS, et al. Ophthalmic presentation of giant cell arteritis in African-Americans. Eye 2017;31(1):113–8.
5. Gonzalez-Gay MA, Miranda-Filloy JA, Lopez-Diaz MJ, et al. Giant cell arteritis in northwestern spain: a 25-year epidemiologic study. Medicine (Baltimore) 2007;86(2):61–8.
6. Liu NH, LaBree LD, Feldon SE, et al. The epidemiology of giant cell arteritis: a 12-year retrospective study. Ophthalmology 2001;108(6):1145–9.
7. Singh AG, Kermani TA, Crowson CS, et al. Visual manifestations in giant cell arteritis: trend over 5 decades in a population-based cohort. J Rheumatol 2015;42(2):309–15.
8. Liu GT, Glaser JS, Schatz NJ, et al. Visual morbidity in giant cell arteritis. Clinical characteristics and prognosis for vision. Ophthalmology 1994;101(11):1779–85.
9. Wilkinson IMS. Arteries of the head and neck in giant cell arteritis: a pathological study to show the pattern of arterial involvement. Arch Neurol 1972;27(5):378.
10. Occult giant cell arteritis: ocular manifestations. Am J Ophthalmol 1998;125(4):521–6.
11. Hayreh SS. Ophthalmic manifestations of giant cell arteritis. In: Hayreh SS, editor. Ischemic optic neuropathies. Berlin, Heidelberg: Springer; 2011. p. 199–226. https://doi.org/10.1007/978-3-642-11852-4_12.
12. Smith JH, Swanson JW. Giant cell arteritis. Headache J Head Face Pain 2014;54(8):1273–89.
13. Ross AG, Jivraj I, Rodriguez G, et al. Retrospective, multicenter comparison of the clinical presentation of patients presenting with diplopia from giant cell arteritis vs other causes. J Neuroophthalmol 2019;39(1):8–13.
14. Giant cell arteritis: validity and reliability of various diagnostic criteria. Am J Ophthalmol 1997;123(3):285–96.
15. Walvick MD, Walvick MP. Giant cell arteritis: laboratory predictors of a positive temporal artery biopsy. Ophthalmology 2011;118(6):1201–4.

16. Foroozan R, Danesh-Meyer H, Savino PJ, et al. Thrombocytosis in patients with biopsy-proven giant cell arteritis. Ophthalmology 2002;109(7):1267–71.
17. Lincoff NS, Erlich PD, Brass LS. Thrombocytosis in temporal arteritis: rising platelet counts: a red flag for giant cell arteritis. J Neuroophthalmol 2000;20(2): 67–72.
18. Giant-cell arteritis and polymyalgia rheumatica | NEJM. New England Journal of Medicine. Available at: https://www-nejm-org.ezproxy.galter.northwestern.edu/doi/10.1056/NEJMcp1214825. Accessed October 21, 2020.
19. Sait MR, Lepore M, Kwasnicki R, et al. The 2016 revised ACR criteria for diagnosis of giant cell arteritis – our case series: can this avoid unnecessary temporal artery biopsies? Int J Surg Open 2017;9:19–23.
20. Jivraj I, Tamhankar M. The treatment of giant cell arteritis. Curr Treat Options Neurol 2017;19(1):2.
21. Arida A, Kyprianou M, Kanakis M, et al. The diagnostic value of ultrasonography-derived edema of the temporal artery wall in giant cell arteritis: a second meta-analysis. BMC Musculoskelet Disord 2010;11:44.
22. Monti S, Floris A, Ponte C, et al. The use of ultrasound to assess giant cell arteritis: review of the current evidence and practical guide for the rheumatologist. Rheumatol Oxf Engl 2018;57(2):227–35.
23. Bley T. Diagnostic value of high-resolution MR imaging in giant cell arteritis. Am J Neuroradiol 2007;28(9):1722–7.
24. Pineles SL, Balcer LJ. Visual loss: optic neuropathies. In: Liu, Volpe, and Galetta's neuro-ophthalmology. 3rd ed. ; 2019:101-196. Available at: https://www-clinicalkey-com.ezproxy.galter.northwestern.edu/#!/content/book/3-s2.0-B97803 23340441000055. Accessed October 21, 2020.
25. Lavi E, Gilden D, Nagel M, et al. Prevalence and distribution of VZV in temporal arteries of patients with giant cell arteritis. Neurology 2015;85(21):1914–5.
26. Johnson LN m d, Arnold AC m d. Incidence of nonarteritic and arteritic anterior ischemic optic neuropathy: population-based study in the state of Missouri and Los Angeles County, California. J Neuroophthalmol 1994;14(1):38–44.
27. Characteristics of patients with nonarteritic anterior ischemic optic neuropathy eligible for the ischemic optic neuropathy decompression trial. Arch Ophthalmol 1996;114(11):1366.
28. Repka MX, Savino PJ, Schatz NJ, et al. Clinical profile and long-term implications of anterior ischemic optic neuropathy. Am J Ophthalmol 1983;96(4):478–83.
29. Hayreh SSM. Role of nocturnal arterial hypotension in nonarteritic anterior ischemic optic neuropathy. [Letter]. J Neuroophthalmol 2017;37(3):350–1.
30. Atkins EJ, Bruce BB, Newman NJ, et al. Treatment of nonarteritic anterior ischemic optic neuropathy. Surv Ophthalmol 2010;55(1):47–63.
31. Aptel F, Khayi H, Pépin J-L, et al. Association of nonarteritic ischemic optic neuropathy with obstructive sleep apnea syndrome: consequences for obstructive sleep apnea screening and treatment. JAMA Ophthalmol 2015;133(7):797.
32. Hayreh SS, Joos KM, Podhajsky PA, et al. Systemic diseases associated with nonarteritic anterior ischemic optic neuropathy. Am J Ophthalmol 1994;118(6): 766–80.
33. O'Sullivan E. Nonarteritic anterior ischemic optic neuropathy and obstructive sleep apnea/a prospective photographic study of the ocular fundus in obstructive sleep apnea. Curr Med Lit Ophthalmol 2013;23(4):143–4.
34. Nonarteritic anterior ischemic optic neuropathy: time of onset of visual loss. Am J Ophthalmol 1997;124(5):641–7.

35. Newman NJ, Scherer R, Langenberg P, et al. The fellow eye in NAION: report from the Ischemic Optic Neuropathy Decompression Trial follow-up study. Am J Ophthalmol 2002;134(3):317–28.

36. The clinical profile of optic neuritis: experience of the optic neuritis treatment trial. Arch Ophthalmol 1991;109(12):1673.

37. Nevalainen J, Krapp E, Paetzold J, et al. Visual field defects in acute optic neuritis - distribution of different types of defect pattern, assessed with threshold-related supraliminal perimetry, ensuring high spatial resolution. Graefes Arch Clin Exp Ophthalmol 2008;246(4):599–607.

38. Keltner JL. Visual field profile of optic neuritis: a final follow-up report from the optic neuritis treatment trial from baseline through 15 years. Arch Ophthalmol 2010; 128(3):330.

39. Fazzone HE, Lefton DR, Kupersmith MJ. Optic neuritis: correlation of pain and magnetic resonance imaging. Ophthalmology 2003;110(8):1646–9.

40. Beck RW. Brain magnetic resonance imaging in acute optic neuritis: experience of the optic neuritis study group. Arch Neurol 1993;50(8):841.

41. Beck RW, Cleary PA, Anderson MM, et al. A randomized, controlled trial of corticosteroids in the treatment of acute optic neuritis. N Engl J Med 1992;326(9): 581–8.

42. Visual function 15 years after optic neuritis: a final follow-up report from the Optic Neuritis Treatment Trial. Ophthalmology 2008;115(6):1079–82.e5.

43. Gout OF. Visual function at baseline and 1 month in acute optic neuritis: predictors of visual outcome. 2020. Available at: https://n-neurology-org.ezproxy.galter. northwestern.edu/content/visual-function-baseline-and-1-month-acute-optic-neuritis-predictors-visual-outcome. Accessed October 22, 2020.

44. MOG-IgG in NMO and related disorders: a multicenter study of 50 patients. Part 1: frequency, syndrome specificity, influence of disease activity, long-term course, association with AQP4-IgG, and origin. In: cooperation with the Neuro-myelitis Optica Study Group (NEMOS), Jarius S, Ruprecht K, et al, editors. J Neuroinflammation 2016;13(1):279.

45. Chen JJ, Tobin WO, Majed M, et al. Prevalence of myelin oligodendrocyte glyco-protein and aquaporin-4–IgG in patients in the Optic Neuritis Treatment Trial. JAMA Ophthalmol 2018;136(4):419.

46. Flanagan EP, Cabre P, Weinshenker BG, et al. Epidemiology of aquaporin-4 auto-immunity and neuromyelitis optica spectrum: aquaporin-4-IgG seroprevalence. Ann Neurol 2016;79(5):775–83.

47. Gobel H. 1.2 Migraine with aura. ICHD-3 The International Classification of Head-ache Disorders 3rd edition. Available at: https://ichd-3.org/1-migraine/1-2-migraine-with-aura/. Accessed October 22, 2020.

48. Evans RW, Grosberg BM. Expert opinion: retinal migraine: migraine associated with monocular visual symptoms (CME). Headache J Head Face Pain 2008; 48(1):142–5.

49. Petzold A, Islam N, Plant GT. Patterns of non-embolic transient monocular visual field loss. J Neurol 2013;260(7):1889–900.

50. Brennan KC, Tang T, Lopez-Valdes H, et al. Minimum conditions for the induction of cortical spreading depression: implications for migraine with Aura (S16.002). Neurology 2012;78(1 Supplement). S16.002-S16.002.

51. Teive HaG, Kowacs PA, Maranhão Filho P, et al. Leao's cortical spreading depres-sion: from experimental "artifact" to physiological principle. Neurology 2005; 65(9):1455–9.

52. An asymmetrical pupil- ClinicalKey. Available at: https://www-clinicalkey-com.
    ezproxy.galter.northwestern.edu/#!/content/playContent/1-s2.0-S0002838X1930
    0474. Accessed September 26, 2020.

53. Balcer LJ. Pupillary disorders, pupillary disorders. In: Liu, Volpe, and Galetta's ;.
    3rd ed. ; 2019:417-447. Available at: https://www-clinicalkey-com.ezproxy.galter.
    northwestern.edu/#!/content/book/3-s2.0-B9780323340441000134. Accessed
    October 22, 2020.

54. Causes of Horner syndrome: a study of 318 patients: Journal of Neuro-Ophthal-
    mology. Available at: https://journals.lww.com/jneuro-ophthalmology/pages/
    articleviewer.aspx?year=2020&issue=09000&article=00012&type=Fulltext&
    fbclid=IwAR3NFrEgpiszf1pJMmGdbBR96nge8ISMICOTFpctZyy3aqylHvoGql-
    6HCE. Accessed October 6, 2020.

55. Wang FM, Wertenbaker C, Cho H, et al. Unilateral straight hair and congenital
    Horner syndrome. J Neuro-Ophthalmol 2012;32(2):132–4.

56. Deprez FC, Coulier J, Rommel D, et al. Congenital Horner syndrome with hetero-
    chromia iridis associated with ipsilateral internal carotid artery hypoplasia. J Clin
    Neurol Seoul Korea 2015;11(2):192–6.

57. Al-Moosa A, Eggenberger E. Neuroimaging yield in isolated Horner syndrome.
    Curr Opin Ophthalmol 2011;22(6):468–71.

58. Mahoney NR, Liu GT, Menacker SJ, et al. Pediatric Horner syndrome: etiologies
    and roles of imaging and urine studies to detect neuroblastoma and other
    responsible mass lesions. Am J Ophthalmol 2006;142(4):651–9.

59. Ksiazek SM, Slamovits TL, Rosen CE, et al. Fascicular arrangement in partial oc-
    ulomotor paresis. Am J Ophthalmol 1994;118(1):97–103.

60. Chaudhary N, Davagnanam I, Ansari SA, et al. Imaging of intracranial aneurysms
    causing isolated third cranial nerve palsy. J Neuro Ophthalmol 2009;29(3):
    238–44.

61. Midbrain syndromes of Benedikt, Claude, and Nothnagel | Neurology. Available
    at: https://n.neurology.org/content/42/9/1820. Accessed September 26, 2020.

62. Foroozan R, Buono LM, Savino PJ, et al. Tonic pupils from giant cell arteritis. Br J
    Ophthalmol 2003;87(4):510–2.

63. Goldstein SM, Liu GT, Edmond JC, et al. Orbital neural-glial hamartoma associ-
    ated with a congenital tonic pupil. J AAPOS 2002;6(1):54–5.

64. Müller NG, Prass K, Zschenderlein R. Anti-Hu antibodies, sensory neuropathy,
    and Holmes-Adie syndrome in a patient with seminoma. Neurology 2005;64(1):
    164–5.

65. Bowie EM, Givre SJ. Tonic pupil and sarcoidosis. Am J Ophthalmol 2003;135(3):
    417–9.

66. Toth C, Fletcher WA. Autonomic disorders and the eye. J Neuro Ophthalmol 2005;
    25(1):1–4.

67. Anzai T, Uematsu D, Takahashi K, et al. Guillain-Barré syndrome with bilateral
    tonic pupils. Intern Med Tokyo Jpn 1994;33(4):248–51.

68. Savitt DL, Roberts JR, Siegel EG. Anisocoria from jimsonweed. JAMA 1986;
    255(11):1439–40.

69. Havelius U, Åsman P. Accidental mydriasis from exposure to Angel's trumpet
    (Datura suaveolens). Acta Ophthalmol Scand 2002;80(3):332–5.

70. Accidental mydriasis from blue nightshade "lipstick". | NOVEL - Journal of Neuro-
    Ophthalmology. Available at: https://collections.lib.utah.edu/details?id=226480.
    Accessed September 26, 2020.

71. Jacobson DM. A prospective evaluation of cholinergic supersensitivity of the iris sphincter in patients with oculomotor nerve palsies. Am J Ophthalmol 1994; 118(3):377–83.
72. Jacobson DM, Vierkant RA. Comparison of cholinergic supersensitivity in third nerve palsy and Adie's syndrome. J Neuroophthalmol 1998;18(3):171–5.
73. De Lott LB, Kerber KA, Lee PP, et al. Diplopia-related ambulatory and emergency department visits in the United States, 2003-2012. JAMA Ophthalmol 2017; 135(12):1339.
74. Comer RM, Dawson E, Plant G, et al. Causes and outcomes for patients presenting with diplopia to an eye casualty department. Eye 2007;21(3):413–8.
75. Nazerian P, Vanni S, Tarocchi C, et al. Causes of diplopia in the emergency department: diagnostic accuracy of clinical assessment and of head computed tomography. Eur J Emerg Med 2014;21(2):118–24.
76. Tamhankar MA. Eye movement disorders: third, fourth, and sixth nerve palsies and other causes of diplopia and ocular misalignment. In: Liu, Volpe, and Galetta's neuro-ophthalmology. 3rd ed. ; 2019:489-547. Available at: https://www-clinicalkey-com.ezproxy.galter.northwestern.edu/#!/content/book/3-s2.0-B97803 23340441000158. Accessed September 19, 2020.
77. Monocular diplopia. [Editorial]. J Clin Neuroophthalmol 1986;6(3):184–5.
78. Barton JJS. "Retinal diplopia" associated with macular wrinkling. Neurology 2004; 63(5):925–7.
79. O'Colmain U, Gilmour C, MacEwEN CJ. Acute-onset diplopia. Acta Ophthalmol 2014;92(4):382–6.
80. Richards BW, Jones FR, Younge BR. Causes and prognosis in 4,278 cases of paralysis of the oculomotor, trochlear, and abducens cranial nerves. Am J Ophthalmol 1992;113(5):489–96.
81. Tamhankar MA, Biousse V, Ying G-S, et al. Isolated third, fourth, and sixth cranial nerve palsies from presumed microvascular versus other causes: a prospective study. Ophthalmology 2013;120(11):2264–9.
82. Tamhankar MA, Volpe NJ. Management of acute cranial nerve 3, 4 and 6 palsies: role of neuroimaging. Curr Opin Ophthalmol 2015;26(6):464–8.
83. Tamhankar MA, Kim JH, Ying G-S, et al. Adult hypertropia: a guide to diagnostic evaluation based on review of 300 patients. Eye 2011;25(1):91–6.
84. Brodsky MC, Donahue SP, Vaphiades M, et al. Skew deviation revisited. Surv Ophthalmol 2006;51(2):105–28.
85. Zee DS. Internuclear ophthalmoplegia: pathophysiology and diagnosis. Baillieres Clin Neurol 1992;1(2):455–70.
86. Kim JS. Internuclear ophthalmoplegia as an isolated or predominant symptom of brainstem infarction. Neurology 2004;62(9):1491–6.
87. Eggenberger E, Golnik K, Lee A, et al. Prognosis of ischemic internuclear ophthalmoplegia. Ophthalmology 2002;109(9):1676–8.
88. Grob D, Arsura EL, Brunner NG, et al. The course of myasthenia gravis and therapies affecting outcome. Ann N Y Acad Sci 1987;505:472–99.
89. Hendricks TM, Bhatti MT, Hodge DO, et al. Incidence, epidemiology, and transformation of ocular myasthenia gravis: a population-based study. Am J Ophthalmol 2019;205:99–105.

# Ocular Oncology—Primary and Metastatic Malignancies

Basil K. Williams Jr, MD[a],*, Maura Di Nicola, MD[b]

## KEYWORDS

- Eye • Intraocular tumor • Conjunctival tumor • Uveal melanoma • Uveal metastasis
- Retinoblastoma • Lymphoma

## KEY POINTS

- Malignant tumors that occur on or in the eye can either originate primarily from the ocular tissues or involve ocular structures secondary to metastatic spread from cancer elsewhere in the body.
- Conjunctival malignancies include ocular surface squamous neoplasia (OSSN), conjunctival melanoma, and conjunctival lymphoma. The prognosis is variable, with OSSN and certain subtypes of lymphoma carrying an excellent prognosis and melanoma potentially a deadly cancer.
- Uveal melanoma is the most common primary intraocular malignancy in adults. Despite successful treatment of the primary lesion, overall prognosis is variable, with metastatic spread occurring in up to 50% of patients.
- Retinoblastoma is the most common intraocular malignancy in children, with high cure rates and greater than 95% survival in high income countries.
- Metastasis reaches the intraocular structures via hematogenous spread, involving primarily the uveal tract. Intraocular metastases originate most commonly from primary cancer of the breast and lung.

## INTRODUCTION

Several malignant processes occur in the eye, either primarily or secondary to a systemic malignancy. Conjunctival tumors can arise from epithelial, melanocytic, and lymphoid cells and include ocular surface squamous neoplasia (OSSN), conjunctival melanoma, and conjunctival lymphoma. Uveal melanoma is the most common primary intraocular malignancy in adults, whereas retinoblastoma (RB) is the most

B.K. Williams is a consultant for Genentech and Castle Biosciences. M. Di Nicola has no financial disclosures.

[a] Ocular Oncology Service, Department of Ophthalmology, University of Cincinnati College of Medicine, 231 Albert Sabin Way, Suite 5415, Cincinnati, OH 45267-0567, USA; [b] Medicine, 231 Albert Sabin Way, Suite 5412, Cincinnati, OH 45267-0567, USA
* Corresponding author.
E-mail address: basilkwilliams@gmail.com
Twitter: @basilkwilliams (B.K.W.); @mauradinicola (M.D.N.)

common in childhood. Intraocular lymphoma occurs rarely and can involve primarily the retina and vitreous or the uveal tract (iris, ciliary body, or choroid). Ocular metastases tend to localize to the uvea most frequently and can be due to a variety of systemic malignancies.

## OCULAR SURFACE SQUAMOUS NEOPLASIA
### Background and Epidemiology

OSSN encompasses epithelial dysplasia, conjunctival intraepithelial neoplasia (CIN), and invasive squamous cell carcinoma,[1] which cannot be differentiated without histopathology. When confined to the surface epithelium (dysplasia or CIN), there is no metastatic potential. Once it penetrates the basement membrane and invades the stroma, however, it can access the lymphatics, potentially metastasizing to regional lymph nodes.[2] The incidence has been reported to range from 0.13 to 1.9 per 100,000, with higher incidence in sun-exposed areas.[1,3,4] Several predisposing factors have been identified, including exposure to ultraviolet light,[4] human papillomavirus,[5] human immunodeficiency virus,[6] cigarette smoke, age, and male sex.[7]

### Clinical Features and Ancillary Testing

OSSN presents as a unilateral, nonpigmented lesion of the interpalpebral conjunctiva at the limbus. It can appear as a fleshy, gelatinous, sessile, or papillomatous mass with varying degree of leukoplakia, dilated feeding vessels, and intrinsic hairpin loop vascularity (**Fig. 1**A, B).[2] With corneal involvement, it appears as a flat, gray, superficial opacity. Patients may complain of irritation, redness, and foreign body sensation.[8]

High-resolution anterior segment (AS)–optical coherence tomography (OCT) has been implemented more recently to confirm the diagnosis or detect recurrence. On AS-OCT, OSSN appears as a thickened, hyper-reflective epithelial lesion, with abrupt transition from normal to abnormal epithelium.[9] Ultrasound biomicroscopy can identify the rare scenario of intraocular invasion.

### Confirmation of Diagnosis

Lesions that can simulate OSSN include pinguecula, pterygium, and conjunctival papilloma (**Fig. 2**).[8] Clinical examination combined with ancillary testing often is sufficient for diagnosis, but histopathology is required for unequivocal confirmation. Excisional biopsy is recommended, unless the lesion is too extensive for complete removal.[2,8] Some investigators have used impression cytology for diagnostic confirmation before surgical removal.[10]

### Treatment

Management of OSSN depends on the extent and location of the tumor. Surgical excision with a 2-mm margin, double freeze-thaw cryotherapy to the margins, and alcohol epitheliectomy for corneal involvement is appropriate for circumscribed disease and offers the advantage of histopathologic confirmation.[2] Multiple topical and intralesional agents have demonstrated adequate tumor control and a favorable side-effect profile, including interferon-α2b and 5-fluorouracil. Mitomycin C also is effective but use as first-line therapy is limited by side effects.[11] Medical therapy is ideal in poor surgical candidates, for cases of extensive corneal involvement, and to reduce recurrence in cases of positive margins after surgical resection. Plaque radiotherapy may be used in refractory or recurrent disease. In rare cases, intraocular or orbital invasion can occur, requiring enucleation (removal of the eye) or exenteration (removal of eye, eyelids, and orbital contents.)

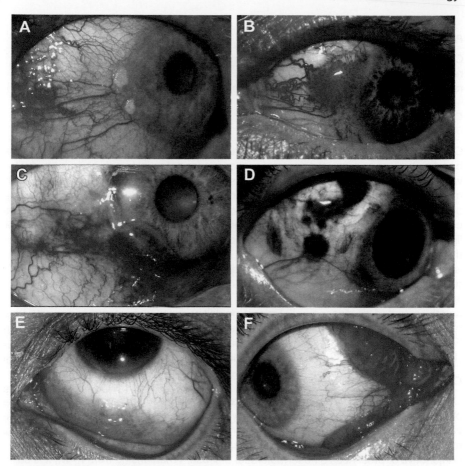

**Fig. 1.** Conjunctival malignancies. OSSN demonstrating typical features, including leukopla-kia with corneal involvement (*A*), dilated feeding vessels, and intrinsic hairpin loop vascu-larity (*B*). Conjunctival melanoma presenting as an elevated amelanotic mass (*C*) and as multifocal, deeply pigmented lesions with surrounding PAM (*D*). Conjunctival lymphoma with typical salmon patch appearance, involving the forniceal (*E*) and bulbar conjunctiva (*F*).

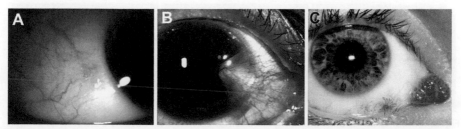

**Fig. 2.** Conjunctival lesions simulating OSSN. Pinguecula is a benign degenerative condition, which usually presents as a slightly elevated white/yellow lesion, most frequently located in the temporal and nasal bulbar conjunctiva (*A*). Pterygium is a surface lesion that tends to originate in the limbal conjunctiva, which presents as an elevated, translucent pinkish lesion with progressive involvement of the cornea (*B*). Conjunctival papilloma appears as a unifo-cal or multifocal elevated pinkish lesion with irregular surface and intrinsic hairpin loop vascularity (*C*).

### Prognosis

OSSN has a favorable prognosis after both surgical and medical treatments, with recurrence rates of 5% and 1% at 1 year, respectively.[7] Lymph node metastasis is rare and occurs in only 1% to 2% of cases.[2]

## CONJUNCTIVAL MELANOMA
### Background and Epidemiology

Conjunctival melanoma is composed of malignant melanocytes that proliferate in the basal epithelium and invade the stroma, allowing for potential lymph node metastasis via lymphatic invasion. Similar to cutaneous melanoma, the incidence of conjunctival melanoma has increased in fair-skinned populations recently and is estimated to occur between 0.2 and 0.8 per million people.[12,13] Conjunctival melanoma is more common in whites and occurs more frequently in middle-aged or elderly men.[13] Sunlight exposure increases risk, but melanoma can occur in nonexposed areas, such as the forniceal and palpebral conjunctiva.[12] Conjunctival melanoma arises from preexisting primary acquired melanosis (PAM), de novo, or conjunctival nevus, in order of decreasing frequency.[14] The risk for conjunctival nevus transformation into melanoma is approximately 1 in 300, whereas the risk for PAM depends on the degree of atypia and the extent of the disease.[15,16] There is no risk of melanoma without atypia, and the rate of transformation into melanoma varies between 12% and 50% with atypia.[16,17] Furthermore, the risk for malignant transformation increases with the extent of PAM (1.7 relative risk for each additional clock hour).[16]

### Clinical Features and Ancillary Testing

Conjunctival melanoma often appears as a circumscribed, pigmented, fleshy, elevated mass on the bulbar conjunctiva, with engorged feeding vessels and intrinsic vascularity. It also can present as an amelanotic variant, making the correct diagnosis more challenging (**Fig. 1**C). Less frequently, it can involve the forniceal and palpebral conjunctiva or present as diffuse/multifocal disease. When arising from PAM, it is surrounded by areas of flat pigmentation (**Fig. 1**D). Corneal invasion can occur, presenting as speckled, superficial pigmentation, often avascular.[2,15] Lesions that can simulate conjunctival melanoma include nevus, complexion-associated melanosis, and PAM (**Fig. 3**).

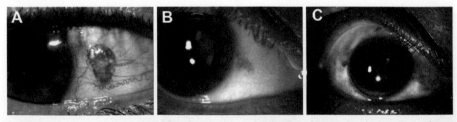

**Fig. 3.** Conjunctival lesions simulating melanoma. Conjunctival nevus is a lesion that often is mildly elevated with variable pigmentation and often is characterized by the presence of cysts and absence of feeding vessels (*A*). PAM appears as a flat area of pigmentation that can appear as pigment dusting. Small areas that have been present and stable for a prolonged period of time generally carry low risk for transformation (*B*). Complexion-associated melanosis occurs in individuals with darker complexion and appears as diffuse flat bilateral, even if asymmetric, conjunctival pigmentation, most prominent at the limbus (*C*).

On AS-OCT, lesions are characterized by hyperreflectivity of the basal epithelium with an underlying subepithelial mass. The absence of cysts helps differentiate conjunctival melanoma from nevus.[18]

### Confirmation of Diagnosis

Diagnosis often is suspected on the basis of clinical presentation, but excisional biopsy for histopathology is the gold standard for diagnosis, and immunohistochemistry rarely is needed. Recent studies focusing on the genetics of conjunctival melanoma have found BRAF mutations to be associated with higher risk for metastasis.[19]

### Treatment

The management of conjunctival melanoma varies based on extent of disease. The mainstay of treatment is surgical resection via a no-touch technique keeping a 2-mm to 3-mm margin and applying double freeze-thaw cryotherapy to the remaining margin.[20] Alcohol epitheliectomy is used for corneal disease. Primary closure may be performed for smaller lesions, whereas an autologous graft or amniotic membrane may be required for closure of larger defects. Initial surgical success is extremely important because the rate of recurrence is higher in cases with positive margins.[14] Rarely, in resistant/recurrent cases, plaque brachytherapy has been used.[21] Lesions that extend into the globe or orbit may require modified enucleation or exenteration. Finally, the use of BRAF inhibitors in patients with BRAF mutation has been investigated in metastatic or unresectable conjunctival melanoma, with encouraging results.[22]

### Prognosis

Conjunctival melanoma recurs locally in up to 50% of cases and metastasizes in 25% to 35% of cases, with overall mortality rates up to 25%.[14] Metastasis may occur in the preauricular or submandibular lymph nodes or in distant organs like the brain, liver, lungs, and skin.[15] For this reason, palpation of lymph nodes is recommended at every visit and periodic systemic surveillance for distant metastasis is warranted. Several clinical features have been associated with higher risk for metastatic spread, including tumor location in the fornix, caruncle, and tarsus. Lesions with positive margins after surgical resection also carry a poorer prognosis.[14]

## CONJUNCTIVAL LYMPHOMA
### Background and Epidemiology

Conjunctival lymphoma is characterized by the proliferation of monomorphic lymphocytes, with varying degrees of anaplasia. In most cases, conjunctival lymphoma is a non-Hodgkin B-cell lymphoma, with extranodal marginal zone lymphoma (EMZL) the most common subtype, followed by follicular lymphoma (FL).[23] It can involve primarily the conjunctiva, or it can be a manifestation of systemic disease. In the latter case, the most common subtypes are diffuse large B-cell lymphoma (DLBCL) and mantle cell lymphoma (MCL).[15,23] Conjunctival lymphoma typically presents in individuals in the sixth or seventh decade of life, with a slight predilection for women in the EMZL type.[23,24] Several predisposing factors have been identified, including infectious/inflammatory conditions and immune system dysregulation.[25]

### Clinical Features and Ancillary Testing

Conjunctival lymphoma presents as a unilateral (less frequently bilateral) fleshy, subepithelial, pink mass, with a smooth or multilobulated surface and mild vascular supply (**Fig. 1**E, F). Due to its appearance, it usually is described as "salmon patch." The most common location is the forniceal or bulbar conjunctiva, and complaints include redness, irritation, and, rarely, ptosis or exophthalmos (in cases of orbital involvement).[26]

Again, AS-OCT has been used to facilitate diagnosis in atypical cases. Conjunctival lymphoma does not involve the epithelium, which therefore appears normal on AS-OCT. It appears as a hyporeflective, homogenous, subepithelial mass with posterior shadowing.[18]

### Confirmation of Diagnosis

Although diagnosis is suspected by clinical appearance, the malignant nature of lymphocytic proliferation is determined only by tissue. Histopathology, immunohistochemistry, flow cytometry, and gene rearrangement studies all can be used to obtain the correct diagnosis. Differential diagnosis includes benign reactive lymphoid hyperplasia, chronic conjunctivitis, and episcleritis.[26]

### Treatment

Once diagnostic confirmation is achieved through biopsy, management of conjunctival lymphoma depends largely on systemic involvement and laterality. Lesions confined to the conjunctiva are treated successfully with external beam radiotherapy (EBRT) in 89% to 100%, with doses ranging between 20 Gy and 30 Gy.[26,27] Alternatives to EBRT include surgical excision and, less frequently, intralesional rituximab.[28] In cases of systemic involvement, chemotherapy and immunotherapy with various regimens are used most commonly.[26]

### Prognosis

Approximately one-third of patients with conjunctival lymphoma have or will develop systemic lymphoma.[29] The rate of systemic disease is 17% for unilateral disease and 47% for bilateral involvement.[29] Systemic evaluation to exclude systemic lymphoma is recommended in all patients at the time of diagnosis. Long-term prognosis is strongly dependent on lymphoma subtype and systemic involvement, with EMZL and FL having an excellent prognosis (survival rates 97% and 82%, respectively), and DLBCL and MCL having poorer prognoses (survival rates 55% and 9%, respectively).[23]

## UVEAL MELANOMA
### Background and Epidemiology

Uveal melanoma is the most common primary malignancy in adults and is reported to be present in 6 to 7 per million in the United States. These tumors arise from melanocytes in the uvea and more commonly develop in patients with predisposing conditions like ocular or oculodermal melanocytosis, BAP1 germline predisposition syndrome, light-colored eyes, and fair skin.[30] Although the prevalence of choroidal nevi is up to 5% of the adult population, malignant transformation of a choroidal nevus to melanoma is rare, less than 1%. Most patients are between 50 years and 70 years old, with rare presentations in childhood.[30] Despite successful treatment of the primary lesion, systemic metastasis occurs in up to 50% of patients, which usually develops through hematogenous spread.[30] Currently, there are not effective therapies for metastatic uveal melanoma, with typically poor responses to chemotherapy and targeted treatments.

### Clinical Features and Ancillary Imaging

More than 90% of uveal melanomas are located in the choroid, with 6% located primarily in the ciliary body and 4% confined to the iris.[31] Iris melanoma may present in a variety of clinical manifestations ranging from small and circumscribed to diffuse and flat (**Fig. 4A**).[32] They may have satellite lesions and cause diffuse angle involvement and can range in pigmentation from primarily transparent to deeply pigmented (**Fig. 4B**). Ciliary body melanoma on the other hand often is obscured by the iris, allowing for the lesions to attain appreciable size before diagnosis. Clinical signs of ciliary body lesions include prominent episcleral (sentinel) vessels, epibulbar pigmentation suggestive of extrascleral extension, secondary glaucoma from angle infiltration, focal cataract, and lens subluxation, among others (**Fig. 4C**). Choroidal melanoma often presents as a dome-shaped or mushroom-shaped mass that may have overlying lipofuscin pigment and an associated exudative detachment (**Fig. 4D**).

Fundus photography highlights the clinical features, discussed previously, and provides documentation of growth over time. Autofluorescence can identify overlying lipofuscin, which clinically can appear orange on pigmented lesions and brown on amelanotic lesions but consistently is hyperautofluorescent (**Fig. 4E**).[33] A-scan and B-scan ultrasonography are among the most helpful imaging modalities for diagnosis of uveal melanoma and for monitoring post-treatment tumor thickness. The lesions commonly present as hollow, dome-shaped or mushroom-shaped lesions that may have an associated exudative retinal detachment, choroidal excavation, and extraocular extension (**Fig. 4F**).[34] On A-scan ultrasonography, the lesions have low to medium internal reflectivity. On enhanced depth imaging (EDI) OCT, melanomas appear as dome-shaped masses that compress the choriocapillaris.[35] OCT, however, is most useful to detect the presence of subtle subretinal fluid to help differentiate melanomas from nevi (**Fig. 4G**). Fluorescein angiography and indocyanine green angiography may

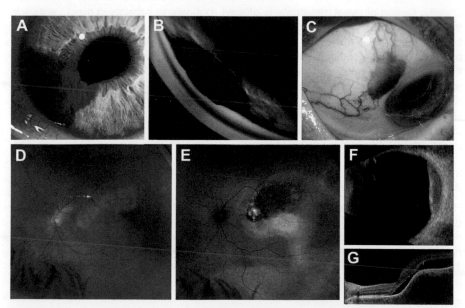

**Fig. 4.** Uveal melanoma. Iris melanoma with corectopia (*A*) and angle involvement on gonioscopy (*B*). Ciliary body melanoma with prominent episcleral vessels and extrascleral extension (*C*). Choroidal melanoma with overlying lipofuscin pigment and subretinal fluid (*D*), appearing hyperautofluorescent on fundus autofluorescence (*E*). B-scan ultrasonography (*F*) and OCT (*G*) of the same choroidal lesion, showing hypoechogenicity and subretinal fluid, respectively.

demonstrate a double circulation for mushroom-shaped melanomas but are most helpful in ruling out other simulating lesions. Globe transillumination helps to identify the dimensions of anterior lesions and can identify ciliary body involvement.

### Treatment

Enucleation was the initial mainstay treatment of uveal melanoma and remains an option for patients with large lesions at risk for extensive radiation complications. Radiotherapy is the most common form of globe-sparing treatment of uveal melanoma worldwide, and plaque brachytherapy is the most utilized form of radiotherapy in the United States. Plaque brachytherapy is a type of treatment that places radioactive seeds close to the tumor. A gold shell containing radioactive seeds is sutured to the sclera, allowing the radiation to treat the tumor across the scleral wall while the gold protects other areas of the body from the radiation. The most common isotopes include iodine-125, ruthenium-106, and palladium-113, and local control is achieved in up to 98% of eyes.[30] Accurately placing plaques on juxtapapillary lesions can be technically more difficult, making proton beam radiotherapy a viable alternative, particularly for these lesions. No direct comparisons have been done between these modalities, but tumor control likely similar is when patient selection is appropriate. Radiation side effects vary depending on the size and location of the tumor and include epithelial keratopathy, cataract formation, scleral necrosis, radiation optic neuropathy, and radiation retinopathy. The visually threatening complications of radiation retinopathy often can be managed with intravitreal injections of antiangiogenic agents or steroids, laser therapy, or residual tumor resection.

### Prognosis

Genetic testing of uveal melanoma is offered routinely to patients in most centers in the United States. Available prognostic techniques offer the possibility of personalized treatment options in the future. A fine-needle aspiration biopsy or vitrector-assisted biopsy may be performed to obtain a tumor sample prior to globe-sparing radiation treatment. Cytogenetic evaluation has shown monosomy 3 or 8q gain increases the risk of metastasis. Gene expression profile testing has analyzed mRNA and categorized patients into class 1 and class 2 tumors, where class 2 tumors are much more likely to metastasize.[30,36] Both techniques are highly accurate and currently are used to identify high-risk patients for systemic metastasis to determine eligibility for prophylactic treatment via clinical trials.

## RETINOBLASTOMA
### Background and Epidemiology

RB is the most common intraocular malignancy in children, with an estimated incidence between 1:16,000 and 1:18,000 live births, resulting in approximately 300 new cases per year in the United States.[37] There is no predilection for ethnicity, race, or sex. The mean age at presentation is 24 months for unilateral cases and 12 months for bilateral cases. Approximately 95% of cases are diagnosed by 5 years of age, but rarely RB can be identified in adulthood.

### Genetics

RB is inherited in a phenotypically autosomal dominant fashion, with 30% to 40% of children having heterozygous germline mutations in the RB tumor suppressor gene located on chromosome 13q14.[38] Approximately 10% of patients with RB have inherited a mutation in the RB1 gene from an affected parent, whereas another 30% of patients have hereditary RB with genetically normal parents, as a result of a de novo event occurring in a single gamete, usually one of the father's sperm. Patients with hereditary RB frequently have bilateral and multifocal disease, an increased risk of pineal gland involvement and second primary malignancies, and a 50% chance of passing the RB1 mutation to an offspring.[38] The remaining 60% of patients develop sporadic RB after having 2 RB1 mutations in a single retinal progenitor or precursor cell. Genetic testing of the affected patient is important to confirm the diagnosis because this changes subsequent surveillance to assess for second primary cancers and for family planning. Testing the biological parents of the affected child also is important to determine the risk of disease development in additional children.

### Clinical Features and Ancillary Testing

The most common findings leading to a diagnosis of RB are leukocoria (white pupillary reflex) and strabismus (**Fig. 5A**).[37] RB varies in presentation based on hereditary status with single lesions in sporadic cases and bilateral and/or multifocal lesions in a majority of germline cases. These tumors are translucent when small and are white or yellow with intrinsic vessels as they enlarge. Additional growth can result in a dilated and tortuous feeding artery and draining vein, intralesional calcification, and an associated retinal detachment. After arising in the retina, the tumor may grow deep toward the subretinal space (exophytic pattern), resulting in subretinal seeds and an exudative detachment. Alternatively, some tumors grow within the retina (endophytic pattern), allowing for seeding to enter the vitreous cavity and in extreme cases to the anterior chamber. Based on the extent of the disease, lesions are categorized in 1 of 5 groups using the International Classification for Intraocular Retinoblastoma (**Fig. 5C–H; Table 1**).

Ancillary testing is valuable in both initial diagnosis and subsequent management of patients with RB. Fundus photography is used to document the clinical examination findings and monitor response to treatment. Fluorescein angiography can be used to highlight feeding arteries, draining veins, and areas of tumor recurrence but is most helpful in identifying vascular complications of chemotherapy or radiation.[39] Ultrasonography is valuable to differentiate RB from simulating lesions by revealing intralesional calcifications, which are present in 95% of RB lesions, and to measure and follow tumor thickness (**Fig. 5B**).[39] OCT can document the intraretinal tumor location for diagnostic confirmation, considering RB appears to originate in the inner nuclear layer.[40] Additionally, OCT can be used during and after treatment of smaller lesions to identify areas of recurrence before they can be detected clinically.[41]

Neuroimaging also plays a role in initial diagnosis and subsequent surveillance. Computed tomography generally is avoided due to the amount of ionizing radiation and the already increased propensity for second primary malignancies.[42] Magnetic resonance imaging provides excellent ocular details and better soft tissue contrast than computed tomography, allowing for more sensitive visualization of optic nerve infiltration.[42] Given the risk of early pineal gland involvement or other intracranial tumors, many centers use magnetic resonance imaging for routine screening every 6 months until the age of 5 years in patients with hereditary disease.

### Treatment

Enucleation was the mainstay of treatment of RB through most of the 1800s and remains a treatment option for advanced, recalcitrant, or recurrent disease. For much of the twentieth century, EBRT became the most common treatment of globe salvage, but local complications and a 3-fold increased rate of second primary malignancies in patients with hereditary disease led to the advent of systemic chemotherapy.[37] Subsequently, EBRT is utilized only as a last resort in patients with multiple recurrences.

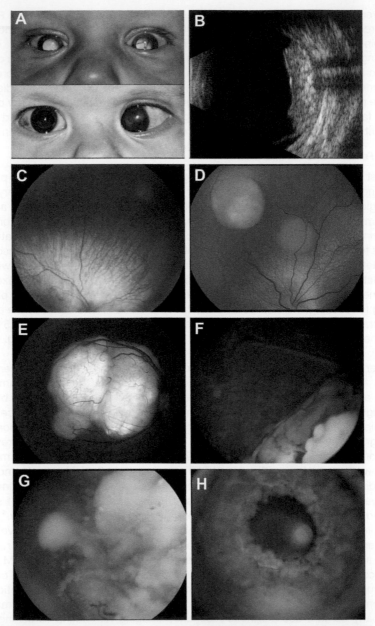

**Fig. 5.** RB. Typical presentations, including leukocoria (*A* [*top*]) and strabismus (*A* [*bottom*]). B-scan ultrasonography of an intraocular mass with calcifications and posterior shadowing (*B*). Multiple presentations of RB: group A (small tumor away from disc and foveola [*C*]), group B (larger tumors confined to the retina [*D*]), group C (large macular tumor with localized subretinal fluid [*E*]), group D (diffuse seeding and subretinal fluid [*F*]), and group E (extensive disease [*G*] with anterior chamber involvement [H]).

**Table 1**
**International Classification for Intraocular Retinoblastoma (Children's Oncology Group)**

| Group | Features |
|---|---|
| A | All tumors are 3 mm or smaller in greatest dimension, confined to the retina<br>All tumors are located further than 3 mm from the foveola and 1.5 mm from the optic disc |
| B | All other tumors confined to the retina not in group A<br>Tumor-associated subretinal fluid <3 mm from the tumor with no subretinal seeding |
| C | Tumor(s) are discrete<br>Subretinal fluid, present or past, without seeding involving up to 1/4 retina<br>Local fine vitreous seeding may be present close to discrete tumor<br>Local subretinal seeding <3 mm (2 DD) from the tumor |
| D | Tumor(s) may be massive or diffuse<br>Subretinal fluid present or past without seeding, involving up to total retinal detachment<br>Diffuse or massive vitreous disease may include "greasy" seeds or avascular tumor masses<br>Diffuse subretinal seeding may include subretinal plaques or tumor nodules |
| E | Tumor touching the lens<br>Tumor anterior to anterior vitreous face involving ciliary body or AS<br>Diffuse infiltrating RB<br>Neovascular glaucoma<br>Opaque media from hemorrhage<br>Tumor necrosis with aseptic orbital cellulites<br>Phthisis bulbi |

Intravenous chemotherapy for intraocular disease became widely utilized in the mid-1990s with a 3-drug core consisting of carboplatin, etoposide, and vincristine. This led to local control in greater than 90% of cases for groups A–C and approximately 50% in group D.[43] Intravenous chemotherapy also is indicated for patients with extraocular RB and as prophylaxis for high risk patients based on pathologic evaluation of enucleation specimens (extensive choroidal invasion, optic nerve involvement extending past the lamina cribrosa, and scleral invasion).[43] Side effects include temporary alopecia, bone marrow suppression, and hearing loss, among others. In order to reduce the risk of systemic side effects and increase the concentration of chemotherapy delivered to the eye, intra-arterial chemotherapy with melphalan alone or some combination of melphalan, carboplatin, and topotecan has been introduced. Administration is performed by catheterization of the ophthalmic artery, after obtaining access through the femoral artery. Intra-arterial chemotherapy has maintained excellent survival rates and can result in globe salvage rates greater than 90%,[44] while significantly reducing the systemic toxicities. Complications, including occlusive vasculopathy and choroidal atrophy, are rare and decrease in frequency with experience.

Intravitreal injections of melphalan and topotecan have increased globe salvage rates in cases of vitreous seeding, which historically has been a cause of treatment failure. Toxicity includes a decreased electroretinography response and retinal atrophy, but long-term visual implications remain to be determined.[45] With appropriate injection techniques, the risk of extraocular seeding is minimal.[46]

Local therapies remain a critical component of the treatment armamentarium for RB and include transpupillary thermotherapy, cryotherapy, and plaque brachytherapy.[43]

Transpupillary thermotherapy provides direct tumor destruction with limited scar expansion. Cryotherapy has the added benefit of disrupting the blood-retina barrier to allow better penetration of chemotherapy but results in larger scar expansion, encouraging use for more peripheral lesions. Plaque brachytherapy provides excellent local control without the increased risk of second primary malignancies. Radiation retinopathy may develop, however, especially in patients previously treated with chemotherapy.

### Prognosis

Prognosis in high-income countries is excellent, with an estimated survival of 95%, but the rate can be as low as 30% in parts of the developing world.[47]

## UVEAL LYMPHOMA
### Background and Epidemiology

Uveal lymphoma is a non-Hodgkin B-cell lymphoma characterized by neoplastic proliferation of lymphoid cells in the uveal tract.[48] The incidence is unknown, but it has been reported to occur more frequently in men around the sixth and seventh decades of life.[49,50] It can be classified as primary uveal lymphoma, when there is no systemic involvement at the time of diagnosis, and secondary uveal lymphoma, when it occurs as an intraocular manifestation of a systemic disease. Primary uveal lymphoma generally is a low-grade lymphoma with an indolent course, with EMZL the most common subtype.[48,49,51] Secondary uveal lymphoma can be a high-grade, more aggressive form, most frequently associated with a systemic diagnosis of diffuse DLBCL.[49,52]

### Clinical Features and Ancillary Testing

The most common symptoms range from painless decrease in vision, to blurred vision, metamorphopsia, photopsia, and rarely pain. Many patients, however, are asymptomatic.[50,53] The most common finding is the presence of unilateral or bilateral choroidal infiltrates that appear as either discrete or multifocal creamy yellow patches at the level of the choroid on fundoscopic examination (**Fig. 6**A). Other rare findings include exudative retinal detachment, choroidal folds, and vitreous haze.[49,53] Iris involvement usually manifests as diffuse, ill-defined iris stromal thickening, with variable degrees of anterior chamber reaction, keratic precipitates, pseudohypopon, and conjunctival injection.[54] The presence of iris and ciliary body involvement tends to be associated with a more aggressive course and systemic disease.[49,54] Uveal

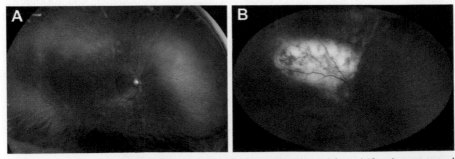

**Fig. 6.** Intraocular lymphoma. Choroidal lymphoma presenting with multifocal, creamy, yellow infiltrates (A). VRL characterized by coalescing pale-yellow sub-RPE deposits and peripheral RPE defects and atrophy (B).

lymphoid infiltration has a tendency to extend through the sclera, manifesting as an epibulbar subconjunctival mass.

The most useful ancillary testing modality is B-scan ultrasonography, which demonstrates a diffuse, hollow, choroidal lesion.[50,53] Indocyanine green angiography is more specific than fluorescein angiography, because it typically shows hypocyanescent lesions corresponding to the areas of choroidal infiltration.[50] Finally, EDI-OCT demonstrates choroidal thickening with a rippled surface.[55]

### Confirmation of Diagnosis

Uveal lymphoma can mimic a variety of conditions, including other neoplasms (choroidal hemangioma, amelanotic choroidal melanoma, and choroidal metastasis) and inflammatory conditions (birdshot chorioretinopathy, sarcoidosis, and scleritis). Given the subtle presentation of this disease, diagnostic delays of several months to years can occur.[50,53] Diagnosis often can be established in the presence of typical clinical and ultrasonographic findings. Biopsy of either epibulbar masses or choroidal infiltrates, however, is required for cytopathology, immunohistochemistry, and flow cytometry to obtain diagnostic confirmation.[49] Systemic work-up is recommended for all patients at the time of diagnosis.

### Treatment

Various management modalities have been considered for uveal lymphoma, including observation, EBRT, systemic chemotherapy, and systemic immunotherapy. Observation can be considered in asymptomatic elderly patients with indolent disease. The most commonly used treatment modality is low-dose EBRT, which allows achievement of complete regression with doses ranging from 1200 Gy to 3600 Gy in a majority of cases.[50,56] Systemic chemotherapy and immunotherapy with rituximab usually are reserved for cases with systemic involvement.

### Prognosis

Prognosis for primary uveal lymphoma is excellent, with high rates of complete regression (72%–79%) after treatment and low rates of recurrence (4%).[50,56] Furthermore, it has been suggested that patients with no previous or concurrent history of systemic lymphoma at the time of ophthalmologic evaluation are at little to no increased risk of development of systemic disease later on in life. In the absence of histopathologic or clinical high-risk features, these patients should undergo annual evaluation by an internist.[53] On the other hand, prognosis for secondary uveal lymphoma tends to be poorer and depends largely on the underlying condition. If high-risk features are present, systemic work-up should be repeated at regular intervals.[53]

### VITREORETINAL LYMPHOMA
#### Background and Epidemiology

Intraocular lymphoma also can affect primarily the retina, vitreous, and optic nerve. This non-Hodgkin DLBCL represents a separate disease entity than the more indolent primary uveal melanoma. The vitreoretinal form is associated closely with and often seen in conjunction with central nervous system (CNS) lymphoma. Although up to 90% of patients who are diagnosed with vitreoretinal lymphoma (VRL) eventually develop CNS disease, only approximately 20% of patients with primary CNS disease develop intraocular involvement.[57,58] The incidence of VRL ranges from 30 cases to 200 cases annually in the United States, but this has been increasing presumably due to increased life expectancy of immunocompromised patients.[57] The median age of diagnosis is 50 years to 60 years, with a seemingly male predilection.[59]

## Clinical Features and Ancillary Testing

There are a variety of presentations of VRL. Some patients experience the vitreous form predominantly, consisting of diffuse vitreous haze with clumps of debris or finer and evenly dispersed cells.[57] Because of the clinical overlap with uveitis and the improvement that can occur with steroids, accurate diagnosis can be delayed. The retinal component presents as pale-yellow sub–retinal pigment epithelium (RPE) deposits that may be multifocal or may coalesce, simulating retinal necrosis (**Fig. 6**B).[59] Later in the disease process, brown clumps of lipofuscin may develop over the lesion, providing a more characteristic appearance and contributing to accurate identification.[57]

Depending on the level of vitreous involvement, wide-field fundus photography can be used to monitor disease progression or response to therapy. Fundus autofluorescence can confirm the presence of overlying lipofuscin, which is brightly hyperautofluorescent, but OCT is the most important ancillary test, because it identifies the sub-RPE location of the pale-yellow deposits.[59] When VRL is suspected, patients should undergo evaluation for CNS disease, including neuroimaging, neurologic evaluation, and possibly lumbar puncture.

## Confirmation of Diagnosis

The average time from VRL symptom onset to diagnosis is 1 year partially because it simulates an infectious or inflammatory conditions and partially because obtaining a tissue diagnosis can be challenging.[59,60] When vitreous disease is present, both nondilute and dilute samples of the vitreous obtained through pars plana vitrectomy are sent for cytopathologic analysis and flow cytometry.[58] In cases without significant vitreous involvement, fine-needle aspiration biopsy of the sub-RPE material may be best. Given the limited volume of these samples, the fragility of the cells, and the sensitivity to corticosteroids, cytopathologic diagnosis can be challenging.[59] Communication with a cytopathologist prior to intervention is key for appropriate transport and rapid evaluation, and consideration should be given to sending out specimens to centers with experience in processing and interpreting these small-volume specimens.

Because of the limitations of cytopathologic diagnosis, additional approaches are being employed. Polymerase chain reaction can be performed to identify monoclonal cell populations and the myeloid differentiation protein MYD88 that is mutated in 60% to 90% of VRL cells in DLBCL.[61] Lastly, cytokine assessment may show an increased interleukin (IL)-10 to IL-6 ratio in cases of lymphoma.[61]

## Treatment

Treatment protocols for VRL vary by site, and the paucity of cases limits the ability to perform randomized controlled trials. Many centers treat patients with VRL and without CNS disease with either intravitreal methotrexate or rituximab or low-dose EBRT.[62] There is evidence, however, suggesting systemic chemotherapy can increase life expectancy when administered at the time of VRL diagnosis alone instead of waiting for CNS disease. Systemic chemotherapy regimens vary, but high-dose methotrexate is the common backbone of therapy. In the setting of concomitant CNS disease and VRL, systemic chemotherapy combined with brain irradiation (including the eyes in the radiation field) may be appropriate.

## Prognosis

Ocular therapy often achieves local control but has limited effect on overall survival, which remains dismal, with progression-free survival over 1 year and overall survival under 3 years.[63]

## UVEAL METASTASIS
### Background and Epidemiology

Metastasis is the most common intraocular malignancy and reaches the intraocular structures via hematogenous spread. As a result, most lesions develop in the uveal tract, and others rarely arise in the retina, vitreous, and optic nerve. It is difficult to ascertain the true incidence of uveal metastasis because peripheral lesions may remain asymptomatic, and patients with extensive disease may have compromised health, preventing presentation to the ophthalmologist. Rates of intraocular metastasis reach as high as 12% historically in the literature,[64] but more recent studies suggest much lower rates,[65] which may be due to improved cancer treatments. Consequently, routine ophthalmic screening in patients with systemic cancer but without visual symptoms is not recommended.[65]

Most cases of uveal metastasis have a known primary, but the ophthalmic findings may be the initial sign of systemic disease in up to one-third of cases.[66] Mean age at diagnosis is 60 with a female predilection.[66] Malignancy most commonly originates from primary cancer of the breast (37%–47% of cases) and lung (20%–27% of cases).[66,67] The remainder is from a diffuse group of primary locations, including the gastrointestinal tract, kidney, and skin, among others. In the approximately 30% of cases that do not have a known primary at the time of uveal metastasis diagnosis, lung carcinoma, pancreatic cancer, and lung carcinoid are the most likely sites of the primary.[66] Despite systemic evaluation, no primary lesion is identified in up to 15% of cases.[66]

### Clinical Features and Ancillary Testing

Intraocular metastasis varies in presentation based on the location of the tumor. The choroid is involved in approximately 90% of cases, and the iris and ciliary body combined comprise most of the remaining 10%.[66] Iris lesions typically appear as single or multiple white, yellow, or pink masses in the stroma. Iris involvement may cause corectopia, dilated intrinsic vessels, scleral or iris feeder vessels, hyphema, ocular hypertension, and rarely iritis or pseudohypopyon.[68] Given their location, ciliary body metastasis is harder to identify clinically and often requires ancillary imaging.

Choroidal lesions most commonly present as unilateral, unifocal amelanotic lesions, with up to 40% located in the macula.[66] Given that macular lesions nearly always are symptomatic, the high rate of macular involvement may be secondary to a larger proportion presenting with visual complaints compared with those with asymptomatic peripheral lesions. Choroidal metastases are often creamy-white or pale-yellow lesions with overlying and/or surrounding subretinal fluid that can be disproportionate compared with uveal melanomas of similar size (**Fig. 7A, B**). They often are low-lying but may have a dome-shaped or multilobulated appearance. Overlying lipofuscin is seen in approximately 80% of cases and appears as brown pigmentation on amelanotic lesions resulting in a leopard spot pattern.[68] Metastatic lesions arising from primary kidney, thyroid, or carcinoid cancer may present with an orange appearance,[66] whereas metastasis from melanoma may cause melanocytic lesions. Skin melanomas have a particular propensity to metastasize to the vitreous. Uveal metastases are bilateral in 20% of cases and multifocal in 20% of cases.[66,67]

Ancillary testing aids in diagnosing choroidal lesions. B-scan ultrasonography demonstrates dense, dome-shaped, or lobulated lesions, with medium to high internal reflectivity on A-scan (**Fig. 7C**). EDI-OCT is useful particularly on smaller lesions, revealing the characteristic lumpy bumpy configuration of the lesion, the compression of the overlying choriocapillaris, and the associated subretinal fluid (**Fig. 7D**).[35]

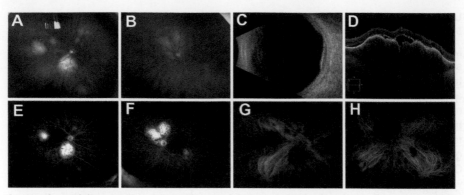

**Fig. 7.** Choroidal metastasis. Bilateral, multifocal metastases appearing as creamy, yellow masses in the right (A) and left eye (B). B-scan ultrasonography of one of the lesions in the right eye, showing medium echogenicity (C). EDI OCT demonstrates the typical lumpy bumpy appearance with associated subretinal fluid (D). The lesions appear hyperfluorescent on fluorescein angiography in the right (E) and left eye (F) and hypocyanescent on indocyanine green angiography in the right (G) and left eye (H).

Fluorescein angiography generally demonstrates early hyperfluorescence with late staining (**Fig. 7**E, F), whereas indocyanine green angiography reveals hypocyanescence (**Fig. 7**G, H). Fundus autofluorescence highlights the overlying lipofuscin pigmentation and pooled fluorophores in subretinal fluid as hyperautofluorescent areas.

### Confirmation of Diagnosis

A majority of patients presenting with intraocular metastasis have a known primary malignancy, but ocular involvement often suggests progression of disease and merits systemic restaging. Additionally, unifocal, amelanotic lesions, in the absence of a known diagnosis of cancer, warrant a full systemic work-up and ultimately may require cytopathologic confirmation and immunohistochemical staining of specimens obtained by fine-needle aspiration biopsy.

### Treatment

Multiple factors assessed in determining the most appropriate treatment include life expectancy, visual function, and patient expectations. Systemic chemotherapy, hormonal therapy, and immunotherapy all have demonstrated reasonable rates of regression of intraocular metastasis. Local treatment, however, is indicated in cases of vision-threatening progression, progression despite systemic therapy, and isolated ophthalmic metastatic disease. Because uveal metastases are radiosensitive, EBRT often is utilized in extensive, multifocal, or bilateral disease. The relatively low dose of radiation (30–50 Gy in multiple fractions) reduces the risk of radiation complications, but the frequency of treatment, especially for patients with advanced disease, is a limiting factor.[69] Plaque brachytherapy achieves excellent success without the need for repeated treatments but typically is reserved for single lesions.[70,71] Photodynamic therapy is less invasive than radiation, can be performed in a single session, and has a success rate of greater than 70%. It is best utilized for amelanotic, smaller, more posterior lesions.[72]

### Prognosis

Even with successful treatment of the ophthalmic metastases, life prognosis remains poor, at less than 25% at 5 years, but survival is linked to the type of primary tumor and to the presence of metastasis in other extraocular sites.[66]

## SUMMARY

Ocular malignant tumors can affect multiple tissues in the eye and have variable presentations. In most cases, diagnosis is achieved through clinical examination, ancillary testing, and cytopathologic/histopathologic evaluation. Referral to an ocular oncology center is recommended to obtain prompt diagnosis and appropriate treatment and follow-up.

## CLINICS CARE POINTS

- When evaluating conjunctival lesions, consider using AS-OCT to aid in the differential diagnosis.

- In patients presenting with conjunctival, uveal, and VRL, perform a systemic evaluation to identify potential disease elsewhere in the body.

- When managing patients with uveal melanoma, consider prognostic testing to evaluate the risk of metastasis.

- In children presenting with leukocoria, in addition to a thorough examination, perform ultrasonography to highlight calcification suggestive of RB. If in doubt, refer to a dedicated pediatric ocular oncology center.

- In patients with ocular metastasis, restage with systemic imaging to determine the most appropriate treatment.

## REFERENCES

1. Lee GA, Hirst LW. Ocular surface squamous neoplasia. Surv Ophthalmol 1995; 39(6):429–50.
2. Shields CL, Shields JA. Tumors of the conjunctiva and cornea. Surv Ophthalmol 2004;49(1):3–24.
3. Al Bayyat G, Arreaza-Kaufman D, Venkateswaran N, et al. Update on pharmacotherapy for ocular surface squamous neoplasia. Eye Vis (Lond) 2019;6:24.
4. Lee GA, Hirst LW. Incidence of ocular surface epithelial dysplasia in metropolitan Brisbane. A 10-year survey. Arch Ophthalmol 1992;110(4):525–7.
5. Scott IU, Karp CL, Nuovo GJ. Human papillomavirus 16 and 18 expression in conjunctival intraepithelial neoplasia. Ophthalmology 2002;109(3):542–7.
6. Guech-Ongey M, Engels EA, Goedert JJ, et al. Elevated risk for squamous cell carcinoma of the conjunctiva among adults with AIDS in the United States. Int J Cancer 2008;122(11):2590–3.
7. Nanji AA, Moon CS, Galor A, et al. Surgical versus medical treatment of ocular surface squamous neoplasia: a comparison of recurrences and complications. Ophthalmology 2014;121(5):994–1000.
8. Maheshwari A, Finger PT. Cancers of the eye. Cancer Metastasis Rev 2018;37(4): 677–90.
9. Thomas BJ, Galor A, Nanji AA, et al. Ultra high-resolution anterior segment optical coherence tomography in the diagnosis and management of ocular surface squamous neoplasia. Ocul Surf 2014;12(1):46–58.
10. Semenova EA, Milman T, Finger PT, et al. The diagnostic value of exfoliative cytology vs histopathology for ocular surface squamous neoplasia. Am J Ophthalmol 2009;148(5):772–8.e1.
11. Nanji AA, Sayyad FE, Karp CL. Topical chemotherapy for ocular surface squamous neoplasia. Curr Opin Ophthalmol 2013;24(4):336–42.

12. Yu GP, Hu DN, McCormick S, et al. Conjunctival melanoma: is it increasing in the United States? Am J Ophthalmol 2003;135(6):800–6.
13. Tuomaala S, Kivelä T. Conjunctival melanoma: is it increasing in the United States? Am J Ophthalmol 2003;136(6):1189–90 [author reply: 1190].
14. Shields CL, Markowitz JS, Belinsky I, et al. Conjunctival melanoma: outcomes based on tumor origin in 382 consecutive cases. Ophthalmology 2011;118(2):389–95.e1-2.
15. Shields CL, Chien JL, Surakiatchanukul T, et al. Conjunctival tumors: review of clinical features, risks, biomarkers, and outcomes. The 2017 J. Donald M. Gass lecture. Asia Pac J Ophthalmol (Phila) 2017;6(2):109–20.
16. Shields JA, Shields CL, Mashayekhi A, et al. Primary acquired melanosis of the conjunctiva: risks for progression to melanoma in 311 eyes. The 2006 Lorenz E. Zimmerman lecture. Ophthalmology 2008;115(3):511–9.e2.
17. Oellers P, Karp CL. Management of pigmented conjunctival lesions. Ocul Surf 2012;10(4):251–63.
18. Nanji AA, Sayyad FE, Galor A, et al. High-resolution optical coherence tomography as an adjunctive tool in the diagnosis of corneal and conjunctival pathology. Ocul Surf 2015;13(3):226–35.
19. Larsen AC, Dahl C, Dahmcke CM, et al. BRAF mutations in conjunctival melanoma: investigation of incidence, clinicopathological features, prognosis and paired premalignant lesions. Acta Ophthalmol 2016;94(5):463–70.
20. Shields JA, Shields CL, De Potter P. Surgical management of circumscribed conjunctival melanomas. Ophthalmic Plast Reconstr Surg 1998;14(3):208–15.
21. Cohen VM, Papastefanou VP, Liu S, et al. The use of strontium-90 Beta radiotherapy as adjuvant treatment for conjunctival melanoma. J Oncol 2013;2013:349162.
22. Mor JM, Heindl LM. Systemic BRAF/MEK inhibitors as a potential treatment option in metastatic conjunctival melanoma. Ocul Oncol Pathol 2017;3(2):133–41.
23. Kirkegaard MM, Rasmussen PK, Coupland SE, et al. Conjunctival lymphoma. An international multicenter retrospective study. JAMA Ophthalmol 2016;134(4):406–14.
24. Coupland SE, Krause L, Delecluse HJ, et al. Lymphoproliferative lesions of the ocular adnexa. Analysis of 112 cases. Ophthalmology 1998;105(8):1430–41.
25. Foster LH, Portell CA. The role of infectious agents, antibiotics, and antiviral therapy in the treatment of extranodal marginal zone lymphoma and other low-grade lymphomas. Curr Treat Options Oncol 2015;16(6):28.
26. Tanenbaum RE, Galor A, Dubovy SR, et al. Classification, diagnosis, and management of conjunctival lymphoma. Eye Vis (Lond) 2019;6:22.
27. Lee GI, Oh D, Kim WS, et al. Low-dose radiation therapy for primary conjunctival marginal zone B-cell lymphoma. Cancer Res Treat 2018;50(2):575–81.
28. Demirci H, Ozgonul C, Diniz Grisolia AB, et al. Intralesional rituximab injection for low-grade conjunctival lymphoma management. Ophthalmology 2020;127(9):1270–3.
29. Shields CL, Shields JA, Carvalho C, et al. Conjunctival lymphoid tumors: clinical analysis of 117 cases and relationship to systemic lymphoma. Ophthalmology 2001;108(5):979–84.
30. Jager MJ, Shields CL, Cebulla CM, et al. Uveal melanoma. Nat Rev Dis Primers 2020;6(1):24.
31. Shields CL, Kaliki S, Furuta M, et al. Clinical spectrum and prognosis of uveal melanoma based on age at presentation in 8,033 cases. Retina 2012;32(7):1363–72.
32. Shields CL, Kaliki S, Hutchinson A, et al. Iris nevus growth into melanoma: analysis of 1611 consecutive eyes: the ABCDEF guide. Ophthalmology 2013;120(4):766–72.

33. Shields CL, Bianciotto C, Pirondini C, et al. Autofluorescence of choroidal melanoma in 51 cases. Br J Ophthalmol 2008;92(5):617–22.
34. Coleman DJ, Silverman RH, Chabi A, et al. High-resolution ultrasonic imaging of the posterior segment. Ophthalmology 2004;111(7):1344–51.
35. Shields CL, Pellegrini M, Ferenczy SR, et al. Enhanced depth imaging optical coherence tomography of intraocular tumors: from placid to seasick to rock and rolling topography. The 2013 Francesco Orzalesi Lecture. Retina 2014; 34(8):1495–512.
36. Dogrusöz M, Jager MJ. Genetic prognostication in uveal melanoma. Acta Ophthalmol 2018;96(4):331–47.
37. Dimaras H, Corson TW, Cobrinik D, et al. Retinoblastoma. Nat Rev Dis Primers 2015;1:15021.
38. Schefler AC, Kim RS. Recent advancements in the management of retinoblastoma and uveal melanoma. F1000Res 2018;7. F1000 Faculty Rev-476.
39. Shields CL, Schoenberg E, Kocher K, et al. Lesions simulating retinoblastoma (pseudoretinoblastoma) in 604 cases: results based on age at presentation. Ophthalmology 2013;120(2):311–6.
40. Welch RJ, Rao R, Gordon PS, et al. Optical coherence tomography of small retinoblastoma. Asia Pac J Ophthalmol (Phila) 2018;7(5):301–6.
41. Soliman SE, VandenHoven C, MacKeen LD, et al. Secondary prevention of retinoblastoma revisited: laser photocoagulation of invisible new retinoblastoma. Ophthalmology 2020;127(1):122–7.
42. Apushkin MA, Apushkin MA, Shapiro MJ, et al. Retinoblastoma and simulating lesions: role of imaging. Neuroimaging Clin N Am 2005;15(1):49–67.
43. Ramasubramanian A, Shields CL. Retinoblastoma. New Delhi, India: Jaypee Brothers, Medical Publishers Pvt. Limited; 2012.
44. Francis JH, Levin AM, Zabor EC, et al. Ten-year experience with ophthalmic artery chemosurgery: ocular and recurrence-free survival. PLoS One 2018;13(5): e0197081.
45. Francis JH, Schaiquevich P, Buitrago E, et al. Local and systemic toxicity of intravitreal melphalan for vitreous seeding in retinoblastoma: a preclinical and clinical study. Ophthalmology 2014;121(9):1810–7.
46. Francis JH, Abramson DH, Ji X, et al. Risk of extraocular extension in eyes with retinoblastoma receiving intravitreous chemotherapy. JAMA Ophthalmol 2017; 135(12):1426–9.
47. Kivelä T. The epidemiological challenge of the most frequent eye cancer: retinoblastoma, an issue of birth and death. Br J Ophthalmol 2009;93(9):1129–31.
48. White VA. Understanding and classification of ocular ymphomas. Ocul Oncol Pathol 2019;5(6):379–86.
49. Coupland SE, Damato B. Understanding intraocular lymphomas. Clin Exp Ophthalmol 2008;36(6):564–78.
50. Aronow ME, Portell CA, Sweetenham JW, et al. Uveal lymphoma: clinical features, diagnostic studies, treatment selection, and outcomes. Ophthalmology 2014; 121(1):334–41.
51. Coupland SE, Foss HD, Hidayat AA, et al. Extranodal marginal zone B cell lymphomas of the uvea: an analysis of 13 cases. J Pathol 2002;197(3):333–40.
52. Valenzuela J, Yeaney GA, Hsi ED, et al. Large B-cell lymphoma of the uvea: Histopathologic variants and clinicopathologic correlation. Surv Ophthalmol 2020; 65(3):361–70.
53. Mashayekhi A, Shukla SY, Shields JA, et al. Choroidal lymphoma: clinical features and association with systemic lymphoma. Ophthalmology 2014;121(1):342–51.

54. Mashayekhi A, Shields CL, Shields JA. Iris involvement by lymphoma: a review of 13 cases. Clin Exp Ophthalmol 2013;41(1):19–26.
55. Shields CL, Arepalli S, Pellegrini M, et al. Choroidal lymphoma shows calm, rippled, or undulating topography on enhanced depth imaging optical coherence tomography in 14 eyes. Retina 2014;34(7):1347–53.
56. Mashayekhi A, Hasanreisoglu M, Shields CL, et al. External beam radiation for choroidal lymphoma: efficacy and complications. Retina 2016;36(10):2006–12.
57. Chan CC, Rubenstein JL, Coupland SE, et al. Primary vitreoretinal lymphoma: a report from an International Primary Central Nervous System Lymphoma Collaborative Group symposium. Oncologist 2011;16(11):1589–99.
58. Coupland SE, Heimann H, Bechrakis NE. Primary intraocular lymphoma: a review of the clinical, histopathological and molecular biological features. Graefes Arch Clin Exp Ophthalmol 2004;242(11):901–13.
59. Takhar JS, Doan TA, Gonzales JA. Primary vitreoretinal lymphoma: empowering our clinical suspicion. Curr Opin Ophthalmol 2019;30(6):491–9.
60. Whitcup SM, de Smet MD, Rubin BI, et al. Intraocular lymphoma. Clinical and histopathologic diagnosis. Ophthalmology 1993;100(9):1399–406.
61. Dawson AC, Williams KA, Appukuttan B, et al. Emerging diagnostic tests for vitreoretinal lymphoma: a review. Clin Exp Ophthalmol 2018;46(8):945–54.
62. Fishburne BC, Wilson DJ, Rosenbaum JT, et al. Intravitreal methotrexate as an adjunctive treatment of intraocular lymphoma. Arch Ophthalmol 1997;115(9):1152–6.
63. Grimm SA, McCannel CA, Omuro AM, et al. Primary CNS lymphoma with intraocular involvement: International PCNSL Collaborative Group Report. Neurology 2008;71(17):1355–60.
64. Bloch RS, Gartner S. The incidence of ocular metastatic carcinoma. Arch Ophthalmol 1971;85(6):673–5.
65. Barak A, Neudorfer M, Heilweil G, et al. Decreased prevalence of asymptomatic choroidal metastasis in disseminated breast and lung cancer: argument against screening. Br J Ophthalmol 2007;91(1):74–5.
66. Welch RJ, Malik K, Mayro EL, et al. Uveal metastasis in 1111 patients: Interval to metastasis and overall survival based on timing of primary cancer diagnosis. Saudi J Ophthalmol 2019;33(3):229–37.
67. Konstantinidis L, Rospond-Kubiak I, Zeolite I, et al. Management of patients with uveal metastases at the Liverpool Ocular Oncology Centre. Br J Ophthalmol 2014;98(1):92–8.
68. Konstantinidis L, Damato B. Intraocular metastases. a review. Asia Pac J Ophthalmol (Phila) 2017;6(2):208–14.
69. Mathis T, Jardel P, Loria O, et al. New concepts in the diagnosis and management of choroidal metastases. Prog Retin Eye Res 2019;68:144–76.
70. Rudoler SB, Corn BW, Shields CL, et al. External beam irradiation for choroid metastases: identification of factors predisposing to long-term sequelae. Int J Radiat Oncol Biol Phys 1997;38(2):251–6.
71. Shields CL. Plaque radiotherapy for the management of uveal metastasis. Curr Opin Ophthalmol 1998;9(3):31–7.
72. Shields CL, Khoo CTL, Mazloumi M, et al. Photodynamic therapy for choroidal metastasis tumor control and visual outcomes in 58 cases: the 2019 Burnier International Ocular Pathology Society lecture. Ophthalmol Retina 2020;4(3):310–9.

# Diseases of the Eyelids and Orbit

Emily Li, MD*, Christopher B. Chambers, MD

## KEYWORDS

- Eyelid • Orbit • Oculoplastic surgery • Thyroid eye disease

## KEY POINTS

- The eyelids and orbit house, protect, and maintain ocular health, enabling normal visual function.
- Common eyelid disorders include lesions and drooping (ptosis). Causes range from benign conditions to life-threatening diseases, the most common of which are included in this article.
- Trauma can affect any portion of the eye and periorbita. The urgency of and need for repair and treatment depend on the severity and extent of injury.

## INTRODUCTION

The human eyelid is a dynamic structure that overlies the orbit, a bony compartment that houses the visual apparatus and supportive soft tissue. Compromise of normal eyelid function can jeopardize ocular health and vision, and orbital disorders can lead to permanent functional deficits. The present article provides an overview of eyelid and orbital anatomy, common disorders, and trauma-related considerations.

## PERIORBITAL ANATOMY

Eyelid anatomy is intricate, dynamic, and exquisitely intertwined with function. The eyelid consists of 7 layers: skin, orbicularis muscle, orbital septum, orbital fat, retractor muscles, tarsus, and conjunctiva. The skin of the eyelid is the thinnest in the body, with no subcutaneous fat.[1,2] Sensory innervation comes from the ophthalmic branch of the trigeminal nerve in the upper eyelid and from the maxillary branch in the lower eyelid.[3] The orbicularis muscle, innervated by the temporal branch of the facial nerve, closes the eyelids. The orbital septum is a fibrous connective tissue layer that extends from the orbital periosteum at the orbital rim to the superior border of the tarsus in the upper eyelid and to the capsulopalpebral fascia just at the border of the tarsus in the lower eyelid. The septum creates an orbital compartment along with the bony walls,

Department of Ophthalmology, University of Washington School of Medicine, Box 359608, 325 9th Avenue, Seattle, WA 98104, USA
* Corresponding author.
E-mail address: emilyli019@gmail.com

Med Clin N Am 105 (2021) 551–562
https://doi.org/10.1016/j.mcna.2021.02.007
0025-7125/21/© 2021 Elsevier Inc. All rights reserved.

enclosing the orbit anteriorly. In the upper eyelid, there are 2 orbital fat pads: medial and central. In the lower eyelid, there are 3: medial, central, and lateral. The inferior oblique muscle runs between the inferior medial and central fat pads. The upper eyelid retractors consist of the levator palpebrae superioris muscle and the superior tarsal muscle, also known as the Muller muscle. The levator muscle is innervated by cranial nerve 3, whereas the sympathetic nervous system innervates the Muller muscle. The analogous structures in the lower eyelid are the capsulopalpebral fascia and the inferior tarsal muscle. The tarsus is a firm connective tissue plate that provides structural support to the eyelids. It measures 10 to 12 mm vertically in the upper eyelid and 4 mm in the lower eyelid; both are approximately 29 mm in horizontal length and 1 mm in thickness. Meibomian glands, which produce the oil component of tears, are embedded within the tarsal plates and open onto the surface of the eye. The conjunctiva is a membranous layer of nonkeratinized squamous epithelium that lines the inner surface of the eye and extends onto the anterior surface of the eyeball as 1 continuous layer that is folded on itself. The conjunctiva contains goblet cells, which secrete the mucin component of tears. The blood supply to the upper eyelid comes from the internal carotid artery, whereas the lower eyelid receives blood from the external carotid artery. The 2 systems have branches that anastomose to form the marginal and peripheral arterial arcades in the eyelid.[1,2] The preseptal venous system drains into the angular vein medially and the superficial temporal vein laterally. Deep to the orbital septum, orbital veins drain into the anterior facial vein and the pterygoid plexus.[2] The lymphatics of the medial upper and lower eyelid drain into the submandibular lymph nodes, whereas the lateral eyelids drain into the preauricular lymph nodes.[1,2]

## CHALAZION/HORDEOLUM

Obstruction of the meibomian glands can lead to focal inflammation and swelling, known as a chalazion. Acutely, the area of inflammation is tender, erythematous, and can be warm to touch. Risk factors include blepharitis and rosacea. Treatment in the acute phase includes warm compresses with digital massage toward the eyelid margin and eyelid hygiene. The focal inflammation is not an infection and does not require antibiotic therapy.[2] Adjuvant management options include oral flaxseed oil supplementation, a short course of topical steroids limited to 2 weeks maximum, topical tea tree oil to the lashes, topical cyclosporine, and oral doxycycline for its antiinflammatory effect.[4–7] The chalazion may open on its own and produce sterile purulent drainage. More invasive treatment options include intraeyelid injection of a steroid or 5-fluorouracil. Risks of steroid injection include depigmentation of the overlying skin and retrograde migration resulting in central retinal artery occlusion, although the latter is extremely rare.[5] A chalazion may require several serial steroid injections to achieve complete resolution. The most aggressive management option is incision and curettage, which consists of eyelid eversion and marsupialization of the chalazion from the posterior surface of the eyelid. This treatment may be combined with a steroid injection, as well.[2,5] Timing of the interventions depends on patient and practitioner preferences. In general, it is reasonable to consider a trial of conservative therapy for 3 to-4 weeks before referral to ophthalmology for further management and possible procedural intervention.

Focal obstruction of the sebaceous meibomian glands can also result in an acute infection, known as a hordeolum or stye. The causative organism is typically a gram-positive bacterium such as *Staphylococcus aureus*. They may resolve with diligent warm compresses and lid hygiene but require systemic antibiotics if they progress to cellulitis. If the inflammation forms an abscess, it typically requires incision and drainage in addition to oral antibiotics.[2,5]

## PREMALIGNANT AND MALIGNANT EYELID TUMORS

Actinic keratosis is the most common precancerous lesion of the skin. It typically presents as a scaly, keratotic plaque on sun-exposed skin in a fair-skinned, elderly patient. The risk of malignant transformation to squamous cell carcinoma (SCC) is 0.24% per year, with up to 25% of actinic keratoses resolving spontaneously over the course of 1 year. Nevertheless, suspected actinic keratosis should undergo biopsy for pathologic confirmation followed by treatment with topical 5-fluorouracil or imiquimod. A patient with multiple actinic keratoses has a 12% to 16% incidence of SCC.[8]

Lentigo maligna is a precancerous lesion consisting of uncontrolled melanocyte proliferation. It appears as a flat area of patchy pigmentation and can be distinguished from benign senile and solar lentigo by its irregular borders, uneven pigmentation, and slow progressive growth. From 30% to 50% of lentigo maligna lesions transform into invasive melanoma. These lesions require complete excision with wide surgical margins and close surveillance for recurrence.[2,9]

Basal cell carcinoma (BCC) accounts for 90% to 95% of eyelid malignancies. It typically occurs in fair-skinned, blue-eyed elderly patients who may already have a history of prior BCCs.

Risk factors include extensive sun exposure in the first 2 decades of life and cigarette smoking. Younger patients may have a systemic syndrome, including basal cell nevus syndrome, also known as Gorlin syndrome, and xeroderma pigmentosa. The most commonly affected periocular location is the lower eyelid (50%–60%), followed by the medial canthus (25%–30%), upper eyelid (15%), and lateral canthus (5%).[2] Clinical presentation varies from chronic eyelid inflammation to a rapidly expanding growth. Nodular BCC is the most common type, appearing as a firm, pearly nodule with telangiectasias and central ulceration. The most aggressive form is morpheaform BCC, which can have poorly defined margins on examination. Clues to malignancy on physical examination include madarosis (loss of eyelashes), ulceration, nonhealing scabbed wounds, and focal chronic inflammation.[10] Incisional or excisional biopsy of suspicious lesions confirms the diagnosis. Treatment is complete surgical excision with clear margins, which may require Mohs micrographic surgery to preserve as much normal eyelid tissue as possible to enable optimal reconstruction.[11] Recurrence, orbital invasion, and metastasis are rare.[10] Extensive disease may require oral vismodegib, a hedgehog pathway inhibitor.[12]

Although SCC is less common than BCC in the periocular region, it is a more aggressive malignancy known for perineural extension, lymphatic spread, and direct invasion. Risk factors include history of prolonged sun exposure, actinic keratosis, and immunodeficiency. SCC that arises from actinic keratosis tends to be less aggressive. Clinical appearance typically includes disruption of normal eyelid architecture, such as madarosis and ulceration. Patients with perineural involvement may report pain. Management and treatment consist of surgical excision with wide margins and pathologic confirmation. Suspicion for orbital invasion or systemic spread warrant further work-up, which may include radiographic imaging and neck dissection with lymph node biopsy.[13] Medical therapy with epidermal growth factor receptor inhibitors, anti–programmed cell death protein 1 (PD-1) antibodies, and hedgehog pathway inhibitors is an alternative treatment option for patients who are poor surgical candidates.[2,14,15] SCC may recur, warranting lifelong surveillance.[13]

Keratoacanthoma is low-grade SCC that occurs in middle-aged and elderly patients, with a higher incidence among those who are immunosuppressed. It presents as a dome-shaped nodule with rolled edges surrounding a central keratin-filled crater.

Although keratoacanthomas can undergo gradual spontaneous resolution, standard treatment is complete surgical excision.[16]

Periocular sebaceous cell adenocarcinoma is a highly malignant tumor of the meibomian glands or accessory sebaceous glands with potential for aggressive local invasion, metastatic spread, and even death. It occurs more commonly in the upper eyelid, where there is a higher concentration of glands compared with the lower eyelid. Sebaceous cell carcinoma affects women more than men and tends to present in patients more than 50 years old.[17] It can occur independently or in association with Muir-Torre syndrome, an autosomal dominant condition characterized by sebaceous neoplasms and colon cancer.[18] Classically, sebaceous cell carcinoma masquerades as chronic or recurrent inflammation, often mistaken for unilateral red eye, unilateral blepharitis, or chalazion recalcitrant to treatment.[17] Recurrent chalazion in the same location or chronic focal inflammation in older patients should raise suspicion for sebaceous cell carcinoma, especially when physical examination reveals madarosis or distortion of normal eyelid architecture. Full-thickness eyelid biopsy with lipid stain on pathology confirms the diagnosis. A map biopsy of the conjunctiva helps to assess the extent of ocular surface spread, given the potential for skip lesions and pagetoid (intraepithelial) spread. Large tumors with suspicion for orbital extension require radiographic imaging. Local treatment consists of wide local excision, possibly with Mohs microsurgery. Tumors that have spread superficially may require adjuvant cryotherapy, and those that have orbital extension require exenteration (surgical removal of the eyeball and all orbital tissue, including periosteum).[17,19] Cases of spread warrant a sentinel lymph node biopsy, as well as systemic work-up for distant metastasis.[20,21]

Cutaneous melanoma is extremely lethal, accounting for greater than 65% of skin cancer deaths, and occurs very rarely on the eyelids.[22] It may arise de novo or transform from a preexisting nevus or lentigo maligna.[22,23] Risk factors include sunlight exposure, genetic predisposition, and environmental exposures.[23,24] New pigmented lesions appearing after the first 2 decades of life should alert suspicion. Features include irregular borders, patchy pigmentation, ulceration, madarosis, and bleeding. The 2 most common types affecting the eyelid are lentigo maligna melanoma and nodular melanoma. The former typically starts as lentigo maligna in the malar skin; a nodular growth arising from the surrounding pigmentation signifies malignant transformation. It can spread superiorly to the eyelid and involve the lid margin and even the conjunctiva. Nodular melanoma is characterized by aggressive vertical spread and may lack pigmentation; there may be deep invasion at the time of diagnosis.[2] Staging is determined by Breslow thickness, Clark level, and ulceration. The most important predictors of survival for localized melanoma include tumor thickness and ulceration. Melanoma with regional lymph node spread carries worse prognosis with a greater number of involved lymph nodes, larger tumor volume, and presence of ulceration. Melanoma with distant metastasis carries a worse prognosis when it involves a visceral anatomic site.[22] Treatment of localized melanoma entails wide local excision with a 5-mm margin, broadened to 10 mm for tumors with Breslow thickness 2 mm or thicker. Thick melanomas (>2 mm) should undergo further work-up with sentinel lymph node biopsy. High-dose radiation is used as adjuvant treatment, as well as therapy for regional lymph node spread and palliative management for metastatic disease. Systemic disease is managed with chemotherapy and immunomodulatory agents.[25] Tumors that are less than 0.75 mm in thickness have a 5-year survival rate as high as 98%, whereas those thicker than 4 mm with ulceration confer a survival rate less than 50%.[26] Local recurrence risk ranges from less than 1% to 25%.[25]

## BLEPHAROPTOSIS

The terms blepharoptosis and ptosis refer to drooping of the upper eyelid, which obstructs incoming light rays and can cause functional visual impairment. Types include myogenic, aponeurotic, neurogenic, and mechanical forms. Levator aponeurosis dehiscence or disinsertion through age-related attenuation, trauma, or repetitive stretching (eye rubbing, contact lens use, eye surgery) is the most common cause of ptosis and warrants surgical evaluation when it impairs activities of daily living.[27] The following discussion focuses on acquired neurogenic and myogenic forms of ptosis with systemic implications.

Neurogenic ptosis results from disruption of innervation to the levator muscle or Muller muscle. Conditions include acquired cranial nerve III palsy, acquired Horner syndrome, and myasthenia gravis. The most common causes of oculomotor nerve palsy are ischemia and compression. Patients with microvascular third nerve palsies typically have a history of diabetes mellitus, atherosclerosis, hypertension, smoking, and associated pain. Examination reveals complete ptosis and restriction of eye adduction, elevation, and depression (down and out).[27] Seventy-five percent of microvascular third nerve palsies spare pupil involvement.[28] Patients with anisocoria with a larger pupil on the involved side, partial third nerve palsy, no microvascular risk factors, age younger than 50 years, and persistent palsy 3 months after onset require neuroimaging to rule out an aneurysmal or neoplastic compressive lesion.[28,29] Patients older than 50 years with concern for giant cell arteritis should undergo immediate serologic work-up, including erythrocyte sedimentation rate, C-reactive protein, platelets, and possible temporal artery biopsy.[28] Horner syndrome results from disruption of sympathetic innervation to the Muller muscle, resulting in mild (2 mm) ptosis and a constricted pupil that does not dilate in dim light. Pharmacologic assessment using apraclonidine or cocaine eyedrops can confirm the diagnosis. The condition requires head, neck, and chest neuroimaging to rule out lethal conditions such as carotid dissection.[28] Myasthenia gravis (MG) is an autoimmune disease caused by autoantibodies to the postsynaptic acetylcholine receptor (AChR) of the neuromuscular junction. It presents as ocular myasthenia without systemic involvement in 20% of cases, but, of these cases, 80% develop systemic symptoms with time. It can involve any ocular striated muscle, including extraocular muscles, which results in diplopia. In patients with ptosis or diplopia that is variable or worse with fatigue, there should be a high level of suspicion for MG.[29,30] Confirmatory testing includes ice test, rest test, single-fiber electromyography, and serologic evaluation for antibodies to AChR and muscle-specific tyrosine kinase (MuSK). From 10% to 20% of patients test negative for AChR; of these, 40% to 70% test positive for anti-MuSK.[29] Patients with MG should undergo chest imaging to assess for highly associated thyroid nodules and thymoma.[28,30]

Acquired myogenic ptosis results from diseases such as chronic progressive external ophthalmoplegia (CPEO), muscular dystrophy, and oculopharyngeal muscular dystrophy.[27,29] CPEO includes a subtype known as Kearns-Sayre syndrome, a mitochondrial disease characterized by bilateral ptosis, progressive limitation in extraocular motility, retinopathy, and heart block.[31] Disease recognition enables potential lifesaving work-up and management.

## ORBITAL ANATOMY

The orbit is a bony cavity that encases the eye and an intricate network of surrounding soft tissue. Seven bones (frontal, maxillary, ethmoid, lacrimal, palatine, and the greater and lesser wings of the sphenoid) form 4 walls arranged to produce a conical space widest anteriorly and tapered at the apex. The septum defines the anterior border of the orbit, creating a closed compartment that is 30 cm³ in volume.[32,33] The bony walls also serve as a barrier between the orbit and the surrounding frontal, ethmoidal, and maxillary sinuses and anterior cranial fossa.[33]

Orbital vessels and nerves pass through several apertures bound by the orbital bones. The superior orbital fissure, formed by the greater and lesser wings of the sphenoid bone, transmits the ocular motor nerves (oculomotor, trochlear, and abducens), branches of the ophthalmic division of the trigeminal nerve (lacrimal, frontal, and nasociliary), a portion of the sympathetic nerve fibers, and the superior ophthalmic vein.[33,34] The inferior orbital fissure communicates the branches of the maxillary division of the trigeminal nerve (infraorbital, zygomatic), the infraorbital artery and vein, the inferior ophthalmic vein, and the parasympathetics to the lacrimal gland. The optic canal, formed by the lesser wing of the sphenoid bone, carries the optic nerve, a portion of the sympathetic nerve fibers, and the ophthalmic artery. The anterior and posterior ethmoidal arteries enter the orbit through the ethmoidal foramina along the frontoethmoidal suture. The zygomaticofacial and zygomaticotemporal canals transmit the zygomatic nerve and vessel branches from the orbit to the temporal fossa and cheek.[33]

The orbital soft tissue protects and enables the eye to function in signal transduction and rotation along 3 axes. The superior oblique and the superior, inferior, lateral, and medial recti muscles originate at the orbital apex; the recti muscles run anteriorly to insert on the globe, forming a muscular cone posterior to the eye. The superior rectus enables elevation, incyclotorsion, and adduction. The inferior rectus facilitates depression, excyclotorsion, and adduction. The medial rectus provides adduction, and the lateral rectus enables abduction. The superior oblique runs in a superomedial direction toward the anterior orbit before it becomes a tendon that attaches at the trochlea; from there, the superior oblique reverses direction to course posterolaterally to insert onto the eye. This pulley system enables incyclotorsion, depression, and abduction. The inferior oblique originates from the maxillary bone periosteum and courses posterotemporally to insert onto the globe. It facilitates excyclotorsion, elevation, and abduction.[33] The oculomotor nerve (cranial nerve III) innervates the superior, medial, and inferior recti. The trochlear nerve (cranial nerve IV) innervates the superior oblique, and the abducens nerve (cranial nerve VI) innervates the lateral rectus.[32,33]

The lacrimal apparatus secretes the aqueous component of tear and provides tear drainage from the ocular surface into the inferior meatus in the nasal cavity. The lacrimal gland, which sits in the superolateral orbit in the lacrimal gland fossa created by the frontal bone, is separated into an orbital lobe and a palpebral lobe by the levator aponeurosis. The aqueous fluid produced by the glands travels in ductules that empty into the superior conjunctival fornix to mix with mucin and oil on the ocular surface.[35] The nasolacrimal drainage system begins at the puncta, which are embedded in the medial margin of each eyelid. Each opens into a canaliculus, which runs medially to the nasolacrimal sac. The sac, located in the lacrimal fossa between the anterior and posterior lacrimal crests, then drains into the nasolacrimal duct. Tears then drain from the duct into the inferior meatus. Contraction of the orbicularis oculi muscle with each blink creates a negative pressure pump system to facilitate tear drainage through the nasolacrimal system.[36]

## ORBITAL EVALUATION

Comprehensive orbital evaluation starts with detailed history intake before a systematic approach to physical examination. The latter includes a focused intraocular evaluation and careful inspection of cranial nerve function, preauricular and submandibular lymph nodes, visual acuity, pupillary reactions, intraocular pressure, extraocular motility, color vision, palpation for resistance to retropulsion, presence or absence of abnormal globe position (proptosis, enophthalmos, hypoglobus, hyperglobus), eyelid position, and visual fields. Measurement of anterior-posterior eye position can be done subjectively by having the patient tilt the head back and looking from the worm's eye view or objectively using an exophthalmometer. Baseline eye position varies among individuals, but asymmetry of greater than 2 mm between the 2 eyes suggests proptosis or enophthalmos of 1 of the 2.[2]

Orbital disease can compromise visual function, lead to permanent blindness, and/ or carry systemic clinical significance. Orbital disorders can manifest from inflammatory, mass effect, structural, vascular, and functional (sensory and/or motor) conditions isolated to the orbit, extending from surrounding structures especially sinuses, or as a manifestation of systemic disease.[2] Anatomic and functional considerations can help to localize the disorder. For example, disease affecting the cavernous sinus can be differentiated from orbital apex lesions by noting normal optic nerve function. Fundamental orbital conditions, including preseptal and orbital cellulitis and thyroid eye disease, are discussed here. Important considerations in the evaluation and management of eyelid and orbital trauma are discussed later.

## CELLULITIS

Infection of the periocular soft tissue ranges from mild preseptal cellulitis to orbital infections with possible intracranial complications. Sources of bacteria include inoculation from skin trauma, direct extension from adjacent structures (sinusitis, dacryocystitis, endophthalmitis, dental infection), and hematologic spread from distant infection. Infection isolated anterior to the orbital septum constitutes preseptal cellulitis and can be treated with oral antibiotics tailored to the bacterial source. Adjuvant therapy includes warm compresses, nasal decongestants for sinusitis, and incision and drainage for abscess collection. Orbital cellulitis requires intravenous antibiotic therapy and close observation for complications such as optic neuropathy, abscess formation, and cavernous sinus thrombosis.[2] Subperiosteal and orbital abscesses may require surgical decompression to control the infection according to evidence-based guidelines established by Garcia and Harris[37]:

- Patient older than 8 years
- Concomitant frontal and/or chronic sinusitis
- Nonmedial location of subperiosteal abscess
- Large subperiosteal abscess
- Anaerobic infection, including infection from odontogenic source
- Recurrence of abscess after previous drainage
- Optic nerve or retinal compromise

Poorly controlled diabetic and immunocompromised patients are at risk for aggressive invasive fungal sinusitis with orbital involvement, which carries high potential to threaten both vision and life. Causative organisms include *Mucor*, *Rhizopus*, and *Aspergillus*.[38,39] Examination typically reveals proptosis, orbital apex syndrome with complete ophthalmoplegia, decreased vision, and necrotic tissue in the nasopharynx. With severely immunosuppressed individuals, such as inpatients receiving chemotherapy, these symptoms may be mild because of lack of an immune response to the fungal infection. Treatment often requires urgent local surgical debridement through transnasal endoscopic decompression and intravenous antifungals.[2,39]

## THYROID EYE DISEASE

Thyroid eye disease (TED), also known as thyroid-associated orbitopathy, thyroid orbitopathy, and Graves ophthalmopathy, is an autoimmune condition characterized by orbital inflammation. Although the exact pathophysiology underlying TED remains partially undefined, research has outlined the mechanism as a loss of immune tolerance to thyroid-stimulating hormone receptor (TSH-R) and insulinlike growth factor-1 receptor (IGF-1R) along with overexpression of IGF-1R. The dysregulation leads to overactivation of orbital fibroblasts, which perpetuate a cascade of orbital inflammation, tissue remodeling, and fibrosis.[40] TED can occur in any state of thyroid function: 90% of patients have Graves hyperthyroidism, 6% are euthyroid, 3% have Hashimoto thyroiditis, and 1% have primary hypothyroidism.[41,42] It affects women 6 times as frequently as men and 7 times more often among smokers compared with nonsmokers.[42,43] Peak incidence is bimodal, occurring among women aged 40 to 44 years and 60 to 64 years and among men aged 45 to 49 years and 65 to 69 years.[41,42]

Active TED is a self-limiting disease that transitions to a chronic inactive phase with a 5% to 10% risk of reactivation. The clinical presentation of active TED varies in severity, ranging from mild dry eyes to severe loss of vision. In mild disease, patients may report foreign body sensation, dry eye, tearing (reflexive), eyelid redness and swelling, eye redness, and spontaneous eye pain. Patients with moderate disease may also notice eyelid retraction, bulging eyes, and possible double vision. Manifestations of severe TED include diplopia, decreased visual acuity and color vision, and loss of visual field in addition to the symptoms of mild and moderate disease.[40–42] Work-up of TED includes full ophthalmic examination, as well as serologic evaluation (thyroid-stimulating hormone, T3, free T4, thyroid-stimulating immunoglobulin, TSH-R antibody, and thyroid peroxidase) and orbital imaging with computed tomography or MRI.[2,43]

Management of TED depends on activity severity. An exception is smoking cessation, which is recommended for all patients.[44] Those with mild disease may be observed or require only supportive therapy, including ocular surface lubrication. For mild to moderate disease, patients may benefit from oral selenium, topical cyclosporine, eyelid taping or moisture chamber goggles overnight, and steroid therapy.[44] Treatment options for active TED causing diplopia and proptosis include oral or intravenous steroids, radiotherapy, and immunomodulatory therapies such as rituximab and tocilizumab.[40] In the chronic phase, patients with persistent proptosis may benefit from orbital decompression, those with strabismus may be managed with prism glasses and/or eye muscle surgery, and patients with eyelid malposition can undergo surgical correction.[43]

## TRAUMA

Periorbital and orbital injuries range from benign contusions to devastating blinding conditions. There may be associated ocular surface and intraocular damage that require a full comprehensive ophthalmologic evaluation to assess (see Cynthia A. Bradford and Andrew T. Melson's article, "Ocular Complaints, Disease and Emergencies in the General Medical Setting," in this issue). The following discussion focuses on the evaluation and management of isolated eyelid and orbital injuries.

## EYELID LACERATION

Penetrating periocular lacerations can extend to any level of depth and can contain retained foreign bodies. If history (projectiles, stab injury, and so forth) and physical evaluation (fat exposure that indicates violation of the orbital septum, visible or palpable embedded foreign body, and so forth) suggest deep injury and/or retained foreign body, computed tomography is indicated for further assessment of the extent of injury. Lacerations that appear isolated to the superficial orbit may extend into the intracranial space. Contaminated wounds require debridement and prophylactic oral antibiotics, especially when the injury violated the septum. Mechanisms of injury that carry a high infection risk, such as dog bites and those involving retained organic matter, also warrant prophylactic antibiotics. Inflammatory foreign bodies typically require urgent removal, whereas inert objects without complications may be observed indefinitely. Orbital foreign bodies that incite acute and chronic inflammatory reactions include organic matter, copper, brass, and bronze. Those that remain relatively inert in the orbit include stone, glass, plastic, steel, and aluminum.[45]

The approach to eyelid laceration repair hinges on whether the injury involves the eyelid margin. Wounds that do not involve the lid margin require only superficial skin closure, even if the laceration violates the orbital septum. Topical ophthalmic antibiotic ointment to the wound helps to prevent exposed tissue from granulating before repair and promotes smooth healing after laceration repair.[45] Injuries that involve the eyelid margin warrant referral to ophthalmology for precise approximation and margin eversion of the wound edges to minimize notching and misalignment.[1,45] Complex wounds also benefit from evaluation by an ophthalmologist to rule out occult vision-threatening injuries, such as globe rupture and retinal detachment.

## CANALICULAR LACERATION

Lacerations that extend medial to the punctum can signify injury to the canaliculus. Canalicular probing performed by an ophthalmologist assesses the extent of injury and can confirm the diagnosis. Canalicular lacerations should undergo repair with silicone stent insertion within 3 to 5 days to minimize the risk of stenosis, which can result in epiphora and need for additional surgery. Patients should be up to date on tetanus status and may benefit from prophylactic oral antibiotics depending on the mechanism of injury.[1,46]

## ORBITAL FRACTURE

Orbital and facial trauma can result in fracture of any wall of the orbit, with or without surrounding soft tissue injury. Patients should undergo ocular examination to rule out concomitant ophthalmic injury even in the setting of blunt trauma and no visual complaints. Emergency sequelae from orbital fractures include retrobulbar hemorrhage causing orbital compartment syndrome, extraocular muscle entrapment, and ocular injuries such as ruptured globe (see Cynthia A. Bradford and Andrew T. Melson's article, "Ocular Complaints, Disease and Emergencies in the General Medical Setting," in this issue).[34] Indications for orbital fracture repair in first few weeks after injury include persistent diplopia in primary and/or downgaze and enophthalmos.[34,47] Large fractures comprising greater than 50% of the floor have a high risk of eventual enophthalmos; however, observation is an option for patients without diplopia and enophthalmos who elect to monitor. Outcomes of surgical repair performed greater than 2 weeks from time of fracture are comparable with those from fracture repair within 2 weeks.[47]

In summary, the eyelids and orbit encompass intricate structures that serve to protect and maintain the function of the visual apparatus. They can present with signs and symptoms of conditions that require urgent testing for life-threatening diseases and/or warrant referral to ophthalmology for further evaluation and management. Early recognition and action by internists and medical subspecialists play a vital role in the management of these periocular conditions.

## CLINICS CARE POINTS

- Signs of eyelid malignancy, including loss of eyelashes, nonhealing ulcers, and recurrent chalazia in the same location, warrant an incisional biopsy or possible referral to an oculoplastic surgery specialist for further evaluation and management.

- Ptosis is a common age-related condition that, nonetheless, may be the presenting symptom of a systemic condition that requires awareness and consideration.

- When evaluating a patient with bilateral proptosis, rule out TED, which is the most common cause of this finding.

- Management of patients with orbital cellulitis includes intravenous antibiotics and close monitoring.

- Patients with eyelid and/or orbital trauma should undergo urgent evaluation and possible repair.

## DISCLOSURE

The authors do not have any commercial or financial conflicts of interest to disclose. E. Li is the endowed James L. Hargiss, MD, Ophthalmic Plastic and Reconstructive Surgery Fellow.

## REFERENCES

1. Cochran ML, Lopez MJ, Czyz CN. Anatomy, head and neck, eyelid. Treasure Island (FL): StatPearls; 2020.
2. Ophthalmology AAO. Basic and clinical science course 2016-2017: orbit, eyelids, and lacrimal system. San Francisco (CA): American Academy Of Ophthalmology; 2016. p. 143–87, 21–26, 43–51, 51–60.
3. Huff T, Daly DT. Neuroanatomy, cranial nerve 5 (trigeminal). Treasure Island (FL): StatPearls; 2020.
4. Yam JC, Tang BS, Chan TM, et al. Ocular demodicidosis as a risk factor of adult recurrent chalazion. Eur J Ophthalmol 2014;24(2):159–63.
5. de la Garza A, Kersten RC, Carter KD. Evaluation and treatment of benign eyelid lesions. In: Ophthalmology AAO, editor. Focal points: clinical modules for ophthalmologists. San Francisco (CA). 2010. p. v. Module 5.
6. Kilic Muftuoglu I, Aydin Akova Y. Clinical findings, follow-up and treatment results in patients with ocular rosacea. Turk J Ophthalmol 2016;46(1):1–6.
7. Jones SM, Weinstein JM, Cumberland P, et al. Visual outcome and corneal changes in children with chronic blepharokeratoconjunctivitis. Ophthalmology 2007;114(12):2271–80.
8. Gupta AK, Davey V, McPhail H. Evaluation of the effectiveness of imiquimod and 5-fluorouracil for the treatment of actinic keratosis: critical review and meta-analysis of efficacy studies. J Cutan Med Surg 2005;9(5):209–14.
9. Mancera N, Smalley KSM, Margo CE. Melanoma of the eyelid and periocular skin: histopathologic classification and molecular pathology. Surv Ophthalmol 2019; 64(3):272–88.

10. Howard GR, Nerad JA, Carter KD, et al. Clinical characteristics associated with orbital invasion of cutaneous basal cell and squamous cell tumors of the eyelid. Am J Ophthalmol 1992;113(2):123–33.

11. Leshin B, Yeatts P, Anscher M, et al. Management of periocular basal cell carcinoma: Mohs' micrographic surgery versus radiotherapy. Surv Ophthalmol 1993; 38(2):193–212.

12. Gill HS, Moscato EE, Chang AL, et al. Vismodegib for periocular and orbital basal cell carcinoma. JAMA Ophthalmol 2013;131(12):1591–4.

13. Reifler DM, Hornblass A. Squamous cell carcinoma of the eyelid. Surv Ophthalmol 1986;30(6):349–65.

14. Gellrich FF, Huning S, Beissert S, et al. Medical treatment of advanced cutaneous squamous-cell carcinoma. J Eur Acad Dermatol Venereol 2019;33(Suppl 8): 38–43.

15. Yin VT, Pfeiffer ML, Esmaeli B. Targeted therapy for orbital and periocular basal cell carcinoma and squamous cell carcinoma. Ophthalmic Plast Reconstr Surg 2013;29(2):87–92.

16. Grossniklaus HE, Wojno TH, Yanoff M, et al. Invasive keratoacanthoma of the eyelid and ocular adnexa. Ophthalmology 1996;103(6):937–41.

17. Shields JA, Demirci H, Marr BP, et al. Sebaceous carcinoma of the eyelids: personal experience with 60 cases. Ophthalmology 2004;111(12):2151–7.

18. Gay JT, Troxell T, Gross GP. Muir-Torre syndrome. Treasure Island (FL): StatPearls; 2020.

19. Khan JA, Doane JF, Grove AS Jr. Sebaceous and meibomian carcinomas of the eyelid. Recognition, diagnosis, and management. Ophthalmic Plast Reconstr Surg 1991;7(1):61–6.

20. Freitag SK, Aakalu VK, Tao JP, et al. Sentinel lymph node biopsy for eyelid and conjunctival malignancy: a report by the American Academy of Ophthalmology. Ophthalmology 2020;127(12):1757–65.

21. Ho VH, Ross MI, Prieto VG, et al. Sentinel lymph node biopsy for sebaceous cell carcinoma and melanoma of the ocular adnexa. Arch Otolaryngol Head Neck Surg 2007;133(8):820–6.

22. Sanchez R, Ivan D, Esmaeli B. Eyelid and periorbital cutaneous malignant melanoma. Int Ophthalmol Clin 2009;49(4):25–43.

23. Boulos PR, Rubin PA. Cutaneous melanomas of the eyelid. Semin Ophthalmol 2006;21(3):195–206.

24. Rastrelli M, Tropea S, Rossi CR, et al. Melanoma: epidemiology, risk factors, pathogenesis, diagnosis and classification. In Vivo 2014;28(6):1005–11.

25. Esmaeli B, Yin VT. Melanoma of the eyelid. In: Wladis EJ, Lauer SA, editors. Clinical education: oculofacial plastic surgery education center. San Francisco (CA): American Academy of Ophthalmology; 2020. p. v.

26. Esmaeli B, Youssef A, Naderi A, et al. Margins of excision for cutaneous melanoma of the eyelid skin: the Collaborative Eyelid Skin Melanoma Group Report. Ophthalmic Plast Reconstr Surg 2003;19(2):96–101.

27. Koka K, Patel BC. Ptosis correction. Treasure Island (FL): StatPearls; 2020.

28. Galtrey CM, Schon F, Nitkunan A. Microvascular non-arteritic ocular motor nerve palsies-what we know and how should we treat? Neuroophthalmology 2015; 39(1):1–11.

29. Latting MW, Huggins AB, Marx DP, et al. Clinical evaluation of blepharoptosis: distinguishing age-related ptosis from masquerade conditions. Semin Plast Surg 2017;31(1):5–16.

30. Gilbert ME, Savino PJ. Ocular myasthenia gravis. Int Ophthalmol Clin 2007;47(4): 93–103, ix.
31. Lee SJ, Na JH, Han J, et al. Ophthalmoplegia in mitochondrial disease. Yonsei Med J 2018;59(10):1190–6.
32. Shumway CL, Motlagh M, Wade M. Anatomy, head and neck, orbit bones. Treasure Island (FL): StatPearls; 2020.
33. Gospe SM, Bhatti MT. Orbital anatomy. Int Ophthalmol Clin 2018;58(2):5–23.
34. Koenen L, Waseem M. Orbital floor (blowout) fracture. Treasure Island (FL): StatPearls; 2020.
35. Machiele R, Lopez MJ, Czyz CN. Anatomy, head and neck, eye lacrimal gland. Treasure Island (FL): StatPearls; 2020.
36. Cochran ML, Aslam S, Czyz CN. Anatomy, head and neck, eye nasolacrimal. Treasure Island (FL): StatPearls; 2020.
37. Garcia GH, Harris GJ. Criteria for nonsurgical management of subperiosteal abscess of the orbit: analysis of outcomes 1988-1998. Ophthalmology 2000;107(8): 1454–6 [discussion: 7–8].
38. Danishyar A, Sergent SR. Orbital cellulitis. Treasure Island (FL): StatPearls; 2020.
39. Hirabayashi KE, Idowu OO, Kalin-Hajdu E, et al. Invasive fungal sinusitis: risk factors for visual acuity outcomes and mortality. Ophthalmic Plast Reconstr Surg 2019;35(6):535–42.
40. Patel A, Yang H, Douglas RS. A new era in the treatment of thyroid eye disease. Am J Ophthalmol 2019;208:281–8.
41. Bartley GB, Fatourechi V, Kadrmas EF, et al. Clinical features of Graves' ophthalmopathy in an incidence cohort. Am J Ophthalmol 1996;121(3):284–90.
42. Bartley GB. The epidemiologic characteristics and clinical course of ophthalmopathy associated with autoimmune thyroid disease in Olmsted County, Minnesota. Trans Am Ophthalmol Soc 1994;92:477–588.
43. Fox TJ, Anastasopoulou C. Graves orbitopathy. Treasure Island (FL): StatPearls; 2020.
44. Dolman PJ, Lucarelli M. Nonsurgical management of thyroid eye disease. San Francisco (CA): Clinical Education: Oculofacial Plastic Surgery Education Center; 2020. p. v.
45. Eyelid laceration. The wills eye manual: office and emergency room diagnosis and treatment of eye disease. Philadelphia: Wolters Kluwer; 2017. p. v, 2020.
46. Rishor-Olney CR, Hinson JW. Canalicular laceration. Treasure Island (FL): StatPearls; 2020.
47. Pelton RW. Orbital floor fractures. In: Clinical education: oculofacial plastic surgery education center. San Francisco (CA): American Academy of Ophthalmology; 2020. p. v.

# Inpatient Ophthalmology Consultations

Dilraj S. Grewal, MD[a],*, Hesham Gabr, MD[a,b]

## KEYWORDS

- Inpatient ophthalmology consultation • Trauma • Hospital • Inpatient • Consultation

## KEY POINTS

- There are important indications for ophthalmic inpatient consults, and it is important for the inpatient primary team to recognize these.
- The authors review the process for obtaining relevant ophthalmic history and conducting a basic ophthalmic examination with measurement of visual acuity for inpatients.
- Indications whereby an ophthalmic consultation should always be obtained are reviewed along with the presenting symptoms. These include patients presenting with sudden decrease of vision, sudden onset of visual field deficit, flashes/floaters, and severe eye pain.

## INTRODUCTION

Comprehensive patient care requires an integrated approach that often includes different specialties. Of these specialties, Ophthalmology stands out with its variable pathologic conditions, unique tools, and special examination techniques, which are often not part of the standard training of internal medicine or other specialties. Consequently, ophthalmology consultation for admitted patients is commonly requested at tertiary hospitals. The consulting team plays an important role in triaging and evaluating the vision problems of their admitted patients. It is imperative for any physician to be familiar with the presentations of the potentially sight-threatening disorders as well as the less acute disorders and the nonurgent eye issues that could be better managed in an outpatient setting. Understanding these different acuity levels helps with delivering appropriate eye care to the inpatients in a timely fashion. In this article, the authors review prior studies focused on inpatient ophthalmology consultations, common reasons for inpatient ophthalmology consultation, and the recommended approach to the most common ocular complaints that could present to the inpatient provider. They also shed light on the basic ocular history and eye examination that should be obtained before requesting an ophthalmic evaluation.

[a] Department of Ophthalmology, Duke University, 2351 Erwin Road, Durham, NC 27705, USA;
[b] Department of Ophthalmology, Ain Shams University, Cairo, Egypt
* Corresponding author.
E-mail address: dilraj.grewal@duke.edu

Med Clin N Am 105 (2021) 563–576
https://doi.org/10.1016/j.mcna.2021.02.006
0025-7125/21/© 2021 Elsevier Inc. All rights reserved.

## INDICATIONS FOR INPATIENT OPHTHALMOLOGY CONSULTATION

There are important indications for ophthalmic inpatient consults to evaluate patients' vision and visual functions. Patients in the hospital may experience aggravation of their preexisting ocular conditions or have a new onset of an ocular problem, for example, pain, redness, and visual loss, or ocular manifestation of their systemic disease. Moreover, the consulting team might ask for ophthalmologic evaluation to rule out certain disorders, such as optic nerve swelling in intracranial hypertension, intraocular infection in endogenous endophthalmitis, or to establish a diagnosis of a suspected genetic syndrome.

Carter and Miller[1] reviewed the Ophthalmology Consultation Service records between July 1990 and January 1997 for 1472 inpatients admitted to University of California Los Angeles Medical Center. Results showed that internal medicine requested the highest percentage of ophthalmology consults (39.7%), followed by surgery (20.9%) and trauma (13.5%). Neurology, psychiatry, pediatrics, and obstetrics and gynecology constituted the remainder. Eye problems were categorized into new eye problems that developed either on the day of admission or during the hospital course, which represented 39.6% of consultations; preexisting eye problems, which represented 31.6%; and screening eye examinations for the remaining 28.7%. Examples of the commonly requested screening examinations were consults to rule out fungal endophthalmitis, diabetic retinopathy, cytomegalovirus retinitis, retinal hemorrhage, papilledema, and requests for assistance with establishing a diagnosis of patients with suspected genetic syndromes that are known to be associated with ocular manifestation, such as glycogen storage disease. There were 92 different reasons for the consults, with the most common reasons being for decreased vision, red eye, ruling out endogenous endophthalmitis, eye pain, and ruling out ocular/orbital trauma. The investigators recorded 166 unique primary ophthalmologic diagnoses and 130 unique secondary ophthalmologic diagnoses. This finding indicates the diverse array of ocular conditions that could be seen in the admitted patients. The most common diagnoses were refractive error, ruled out endogenous endophthalmitis, conjunctivitis, diabetic retinopathy, and corneal abrasion. These data suggested that refractive error is an important cause for decreased vision in admitted patients. The most common primary hospital discharge diagnoses at that time was human immunodeficiency virus infection (HIV), which, despite being the most prevalent diagnosis, represented only 1.6% of the overall consults to ophthalmology, followed by acute myeloid leukemia (1.6%), liver cirrhosis, postoperative infection, complications of bone marrow transplantation, and infection or inflammatory reaction owing to an internal prosthetic device, implant, or graft. There were other 947 different or unique primary discharge diagnoses, which makes it difficult to predict the most susceptible patient population to have eye issues during their hospital stay.

The authors' group reviewed the electronic medical records of 974 inpatient ophthalmology consultations performed from October 2007 to October 2011 at Northwestern Memorial Hospital in Chicago.[2] The most common reasons for ophthalmology consultation in this study were blurred vision, trauma, or orbital fracture on computed tomographic (CT) scan, red eye, eye pain, and to rule out endogenous endophthalmitis. These results were in accordance with the findings reported by Carter and Miller[1] conducted 20 years before. This study also showed that input from the ophthalmology consult service influenced the management plan in 56.5% of consults. The ophthalmology consult service recommended initiation of topical ocular medication in 324 patients (33.3%). Systemic medications were recommended by ophthalmology in 75 patients (7.7%); neuroimaging was ordered in 41 (4.2%), and laboratory investigations were recommended in 13 (1.3%).

Oh and colleagues[3] recently reviewed data obtained from 581 ophthalmology consultations requested at the University of Illinois Hospital over a 1-year period from the inpatient teams (59.4%) and the Emergency Department team (40.6%). The most common inpatient consulting services were internal medicine (21.5%), followed by neurosurgery (16.2%) and neurology (7.4%). Reasons for consultation were divided into 10 categories. Most commonly were vision changes (30.3%), followed by eye pain (19.8%), and periorbital pain and swelling (12.0%). Other categories included trauma (10.0%), papilledema (8.4%), tumor (4.8%), ruling out ocular involvement in fungemia (4.8%), syndromic evaluation (4.0%), optic neuritis (1.4%), and others (4.5%). Consultations were categorized as acute (72.3%), which indicates new eye issues that either prompted the patients to go the emergency department or developed during their hospital course; preexisting ocular conditions (6.0%); or screening (21.7%). Screening consultations were further classified into the following categories: papilledema (31.0%), to rule out ocular involvement in fungemia (20.6%), syndromic evaluation (19.8%), visual field assessment (17.5%), and miscellaneous evaluation (11.1%). Positive ocular findings were observed in none of fungemia consultations, 20.5% of papilledema consultations, 52.0% of syndromic consultations, 27.3% of visual field consultations, and 14.3% of miscellaneous consultations. The study recorded 63 different primary ocular diagnoses and classified them based on the ophthalmology subspecialty with the most common ones being cornea/external disease (18%, common diagnosis dry eye, corneal abrasion, subconjunctival hemorrhage, conjunctivitis, corneal ulcer, and hyphema), neuroophthalmology (17.2%, common diagnosis optic neuritis, cranial nerve palsy, optic neuropathy, papilledema screening, visual field defect screening, and cerebrovascular accident), and orbit/oculoplastics (16.3%, common diagnosis orbital wall fracture, preseptal and orbital cellulitis).

These large studies demonstrated that vision changes, eye pain, red eye, orbital trauma, and screening eye examinations to rule out or confirm a certain diagnosis are among the most common reasons for ophthalmology consultation in the inpatient setting. Although the ophthalmology consult team is responsible for the comprehensive evaluation and final management of all the inpatients with eye-related disorders, the inpatient primary team has an important role in triaging the acuity of the ocular disorder and determining the need for an urgent ophthalmic consultation versus scheduling an outpatient follow-up examination.

## BEFORE REQUESTING AN INPATIENT OPHTHALMIC CONSULTATION

The ophthalmology consult service usually receives multiple consults per day, and triaging the acuity of each consult is helpful for optimum and efficient patient care. The primary inpatient team plays a pivotal role in assisting the different consult services, and it is important for the inpatient practitioner to be able to obtain relevant history and perform a basic eye examination before discussing the case with the ophthalmology service.

## HISTORY

It is important to collect pertinent information to help assess the level of acuity of the patient's complaint and narrow down the differential diagnosis. This history includes information about severity of the presenting complaint, laterality (unilateral vs bilateral), onset (sudden/acute vs gradual), course (progressive vs stationary), duration (seconds, minutes, hours, days, months, or years), history of prior similar episodes, history of refractive error (wearing eyeglasses), and chronic eye disease, such as glaucoma or macular degeneration. History should also include any possible source of eye trauma during or before the hospital stay, such as an unwitnessed fall. It is also important to ask about any other associated symptoms, such as nausea, vomiting, headache, fever, focal weakness, paresthesia, joint or muscle pain, headache, auras preceding migraines, flashes of light or floaters, and double vision.

## EYE EXAMINATION

The basic eye examination is divided into 6 main parts: visual acuity, visual field, pupils, movement of extraocular muscle, anterior segment with intraocular pressure assessment, and posterior segment examination. Although a detailed examination of the anterior and posterior segment needs specific equipment that might not be available to the inpatient team, other parts of the eye examination should be performed for each patient with any eye complaint. Gross external eye inspection under good illumination using a penlight can also provide the inpatient team with useful information, such as THE presence of eyelid swelling, conjunctival redness, and corneal foreign body.

## VISUAL ACUITY

Visual acuity should be tested 1 eye at a time, with glasses or contact lenses in place if the patient usually wears them. In the inpatient setting, near visual acuity is usually tested using a handheld visual acuity card placed at a normal reading distance, which is usually 40 cm from the patient. Each line on the near acuity card is equivalent to a certain distant acuity that is written on the card next to that specific line. If the patient is unable to read any of the figures on the card, the patient is asked to count the fingers on the examiner's hand, and the distance at which the patient can count fingers is determined. If the patient cannot count fingers, then the ability to detect hand motion is evaluated. For this, the patient's opposite eye is occluded, and a light source is directed from behind the patient to the examiner's hand that is moved at 1 motion per second at a distance of 60 cm from the eye. The patient is asked to identify whether the examiner's hand was still or moving. If the patient is unable to detect hand movements, the examiner should determine whether the patient can perceive light or not, with the light source set at maximum intensity.

## VISUAL FIELD

Vision changes associated with acute visual field defects can narrow down the differential diagnosis to disorders affecting mainly the retina or visual pathway. Examples include retinal detachment,[4] neurologic diseases, such as cerebrovascular accident, or neuroophthalmologic diseases, such as anterior ischemic optic neuropathy.[5] The confrontation visual field test is a simple and quick method to test the 4 quadrants (superior, nasal, inferior, and temporal) of the peripheral vision to identify visual field defects. The test is done in a face-to-face position at about 1 m (3 feet). With each eye tested separately, the patient's responses are compared with the normal visual field of the examiner in the superior, inferior, nasal, and temporal quadrants. This simple test can be of a high yield in identifying homonymous field defects associated with cerebrovascular accidents affecting occipital, parietal, or temporal lobes, altitudinal field defect associated with anterior ischemic optic neuropathy, and quadratic or hemispheric defects associated with retinal detachments.

## PUPILS

The pupils should be round, symmetric, regular, equal in size in dark and light, and reactive to light. Pupils examination should be performed in a dim light with patients fixating their eyes on a distant object.[6] An afferent pupillary defect (paradoxic pupillary dilatation in response to light) is an important sign of unilateral or bilateral asymmetric optic nerve disease, such as optic neuritis and ischemic optic neuropathy or severe retinal disorder.[7] It is also important to recognize that certain medications, such as a scopolamine patch, may cause pharmacologic pupil dilation.

## OCULAR MOTILITY EXAMINATION

Ideally, ocular motility is tested by first detecting the eye position in the primary gaze and then asking the patient to move their eyes in 8 positions (up, right, up right, down right, down, left, up left, and down left). This test should be performed for each eye separately and then with both eyes. Testing in the 4 cardinal positions (up, down, right, and left) is also acceptable as a quick screening test for ocular misalignment.[8] The extraocular muscles should work in harmony, and eye movements should be smooth, symmetric, and with no restriction. Ocular motility examination is particularly important in cases with facial and orbital trauma. Patients may sometimes describe diplopia as blurred vision.

## ANTERIOR SEGMENT

The anterior segment of the eye is formed of the sclera, conjunctiva, cornea, anterior chamber, iris, and lens. The examiner can use simple illumination with a penlight to screen and inspect the structures of the anterior segment. The sclera and conjunctiva should be examined for discharge and vascular injection. The cornea should be examined for clarity, transparency, and luster (sheen). Corneal opacification or loss of luster may indicate a corneal pathologic condition, such as corneal ulcer. The anterior chamber is the space between the cornea and the iris that is filled with clear aqueous humor. This space can be filled with hypopyon (pus) in cases of infections, such as endogenous endophthalmitis, or with blood (hyphema) in cases following trauma or with neovascularization.[9]

## POSTERIOR SEGMENT

The posterior segment includes the vitreous, the retina, and the optic nerve, and evaluation requires certain skills and special tools (indirect ophthalmoscopy and a 20- or 28 D lens) that are usually used by the ophthalmologist. However, if the practitioner feels comfortable with using the direct ophthalmoscope, they can obtain important information about the posterior segment. Examples include evaluation of the red reflex, which can be abnormal in certain cases, such as retinal detachment and vitreous hemorrhage. Moreover, the optic nerve head can also be evaluated, which normally appears flat with well-defined edges. The background of the fundus view by the direct ophthalmoscopy represents the retina, which is normally flat and without hemorrhages or exudates.[8] Dilation of the pupil by eye drops facilitates examination of the posterior segment; however, it should usually be performed after discussion with the ophthalmology team.

After obtaining a history and performing a basic eye examination, the inpatient team should be able to triage the patient's ocular condition and obtain pertinent information so that a differential diagnosis can be formulated that is helpful to determine the need for an urgent ophthalmic evaluation.

In the following section of this article, the authors discuss the differential diagnoses of the common reasons for ophthalmology consultation as well as other less common but important reasons for requesting ophthalmology evaluation for an admitted patient. They also shed light on the recommended approach for evaluating these complaints by the inpatient team.

## DIFFERENTIAL DIAGNOSES AND APPROACH TO COMMON REASONS FOR INPATIENT OPHTHALMOLOGY CONSULTATION
### Vision Changes/Blurred Vision/Loss of Vision

Blurred vision is considered the most common reported ophthalmic complaint.[8] It is a broad complaint that can present in multiple ways and has a wide range of differential diagnoses with variable levels of acuity.

### Causes of blurred vision

As discussed above, history taking and a basic eye examination can help triage the acuity of the vision changes and the need for urgent inpatient ophthalmology consultation. It is helpful to have a diagnostic approach for the common causes of blurred/ decreased/loss of vision in the inpatient based on the onset (sudden/acute vs gradual), laterality (unilateral vs bilateral), duration (seconds, minutes, hours, days, months), and the presence or absence of pain.

**Transient visual loss.** Transient visual loss (TVL) usually presents as sudden painless vision loss (vision returns to normal within 24 hours, usually within 1 hour). Unilateral or more commonly bilateral TVL that occurs for a few seconds and often triggered by postural changes is usually seen with papilledema.[10] Patients with papilledema might also complain of headache, nausea, vomiting, tinnitus, and diplopia. Unilateral TVL that occurs for a few minutes is typically seen with amaurosis fugax, which may be indicative of retinal or optic nerve ischemia secondary to a thrombotic vascular cause, such carotid artery stenosis, an embolic source, such as valvular heart disease, or vasculitis, as in giant cell arteritis (GCA).[11] Consequently, a stroke work up and obtaining history about GCA symptoms are important in these patients. It is also helpful to obtain a complete blood count with platelets, erythrocyte sedimentation rate, and C-reactive protein in suspected GCA cases. Stroke work up is warranted in bilateral TVL that lasts for a few minutes, as this might indicate vertebrobasilar insufficiency.[12] If TVL lasts between 10 and 60 minutes, a retinal migraine may be suspected, which is a TVL in the setting of a typical migraine.[13] Inpatient ophthalmology consultation is warranted in these cases to rule out other less common causes of TVL, including an impending central vein occlusion, central retinal artery occlusion, optic disc drusen, angle closure glaucoma, and ocular ischemic syndrome.[11]

### Visual loss lasting greater than 24 hours

**Sudden, painless loss of vision** Sudden, unilateral, persistent, painless loss of vision often results from disorders in the posterior segment of the eye. Common causes include vitreous hemorrhage more commonly associated with diabetes or trauma,[14] retinal detachment, central retinal artery or vein occlusion, anterior ischemic optic neuropathy (arteritic as in GCA, or nonarteritic ischemic optic neuropathy). Urgent inpatient ophthalmologic consultation should be requested in case any of these disorders is suspected.[15] Also, it is important to note that cerebrovascular accidents affecting the retro-chiasmal visual pathway can cause bilateral vision loss in the form of a homonymous hemianopic or quadrantanopic field defect. However, this field deficit is usually interpreted by the patient as a unilateral vision loss in the affected side of the field deficit. For example, a right hemianopia could be perceived by the patient as right monocular vision loss, as patients often are unable to appreciate their nasal field deficit and only notice their temporal field deficit.[11]

**Sudden, unilateral, painful loss of vision** Common causes are acute angle closure glaucoma, uveitis (usually also associated with light sensitivity), endophthalmitis, keratitis, corneal ulcer, optic neuritis (usually in younger patients, associated with pain with eye movements), and orbital cellulitis. Urgent evaluation by ophthalmology is needed in these cases.[15]

**Gradual, unilateral, or bilateral, painless loss of vision (over weeks, months, or years)** Common causes include refractive error, cataract, open angle or chronic angle closure glaucoma, chronic retinal disorders, such as age-related macular degeneration and diabetic retinopathy. Outpatient referral to ophthalmology is recommended in these cases.[8]

Less common causes that require outpatient monitoring by ophthalmology are conditions caused by ocular toxicity of certain medications, such hydroxychloroquine and ethambutol.[16]

## CLINICS CARE POINTS

- Acute vision loss can be transient vision loss (vision returns to normal within 24 hours, usually within 1 hour) or persistent (lasting more than 24 hours).

- Transient vision loss that lasts for a few seconds (more with postural changes) can be seen in papilledema, more commonly bilateral.

- Amaurosis fugax is a unilateral painless transient vision loss that occurs for a few minutes and indicates retinal or optic nerve ischemia secondary to a thrombotic, embolic, or inflammatory vascular cause. Obtain stroke work up and rule out giant cell arteritis by careful history, erythrocyte sedimentation rate, and C-reactive protein. Vertebrobasilar insufficiency can present with bilateral transient vision loss.

- Acute persistent, painless loss of vision is an indication for an urgent ophthalmic evaluation to rule out certain retinal and optic nerve disorders. Stroke work up should be obtained if the ophthalmology team ruled out an ocular cause or the patient has additional neurologic symptoms.

- Acute persistent, painful loss of vision is an indication for an urgent ophthalmic evaluation to rule out certain sight-threatening disorders, such as acute angle closure glaucoma, uveitis, endophthalmitis, keratitis, corneal ulcer, optic neuritis, and orbital cellulitis.

- It should be pointed out that certain surgical interventions could be complicated by vision loss in the immediate postoperative period, such as cardiac catheterization owing to distal spread of emboli resulting in central retinal artery occlusion,[17] and endoscopic sinus surgery.[18]

### Red Eye

Red eye is a common presenting symptom in the inpatient setting.[1–3] Examples include subconjunctival hemorrhage, corneal abrasions, most cases of conjunctivitis, and blepharitis.[19,20] In **Table 1**, the authors briefly review the differential diagnosis and approach to red eye, focusing mainly on the conditions that warrant an urgent ophthalmology consultation.

### Eye Pain

Common causes of eye pain are conjunctivitis, dry eye, corneal abrasion, and hordeolum, which can often be managed by the primary care team.[30] It is estimated in some studies[31,32] that these conditions constitute more than 50% of all eye problems. Most of the ocular conditions that present with eye pain usually originate from the anterior

**Table 1**
Ocular conditions presenting with eye redness that require urgent inpatient ophthalmology consultation

| Condition | History | Symptoms | Signs |
|---|---|---|---|
| Episcleritis | Usually idiopathic but may be associated with autoimmune disorders in 25%–30% of cases[21,22] | • Mild to moderate eye pain<br>• Vision is usually intact | Focal or diffuse conjunctival and episcleral injection of blood vessels |
| Scleritis | May be the first sign of an autoimmune disorder in 30%–50% of cases[23] | • Moderate to severe eye pain<br>• Vision might be reduced | Focal or diffuse conjunctival and episcleral injection of blood vessels, usually at a deeper level than episcleritis |
| Keratitis/corneal ulcer | Contact lens wear, immunosuppression, eye trauma, and corneal abrasion.[24] History of prior herpetic keratitis | • Photophobia, moderate to severe eye pain<br>• Reduced vision | Abnormal corneal light reflex, loss of corneal luster and transparency, corneal opacity, and conjunctival injection |
| Anterior uveitis/iritis | Prior episodes of anterior uveitis and associated autoimmune disorders, such as ankylosing spondylitis[25] | • Eye pain and photophobia<br>• Normal or reduced vision | Circumcorneal injection of blood vessels, ± irregular pupil |
| Acute angle-closure glaucoma | History of angle closure glaucoma or prior episodes of acute angle closure glaucoma, hyperopia | • Severe eye pain, photophobia<br>• Reduced vision<br>• ± Headache, nausea, and vomiting | Circumcorneal injection of blood vessels, hazy cornea, middilated nonreactive pupil |
| Endogenous endophthalmitis[a] | Bacteremia/fungemia in patients with diabetes mellitus, urinary tract infection, immunosuppression (especially associated with underlying malignancy, neutropenia, and HIV), intravenous drug abuse, and indwelling catheters[26] | • Severe eye pain<br>• Marked reduction of vision | Diffuse conjunctival injection ± hypopyon in the anterior chamber ± corneal haze |

| Orbital cellulitis[a] | History of sinus disease[27] | |
| --- | --- | --- |
| • Periocular pain, pain with eye movement, and swelling of upper and lower eyelids<br>• Normal or reduced vision | | • Tender swollen eyelids<br>• Diffuse conjunctival injection with conjunctival chemosis<br>• Limited extraocular muscle movement<br>• Proptosis<br>• ± Relative afferent pupillary defect in severe cases |

[a] It is important to note that immunocompromised patients have difficulty in mounting an immune response, so symptoms of orbital cellulitis[28] and endophthalmitis[29] might be very mild. Higher index of suspicion and lower threshold for consulting ophthalmology, even with mild symptoms, are recommended in these cases.

*Data from Refs. [21-29]*

segment or ocular adnexa and in many cases are associated with red eye.[30] One important exception to the commonly associated eye redness with eye pain is optic neuritis, which usually presents with eye pain, pain with eye movement, reduced vision, and no eye redness.[33]

New onset of dry eye symptoms (eg, eye pain, gritty or foreign body sensation, with or without eye redness) after hematopoietic stem cell transplantation could be an early manifestation of graft-versus-host disease.[34] There are also certain classes of chemotherapy medications, such as MEK inhibitors, that can cause inflammation or blurred vision, and these warrant an ophthalmic consultation.

## Flashes and Floaters

Flashes of light (photopsia) refer to the perception of streaks or spots of light in the absence of external light stimuli. Flashes can be a symptom of vitreoretinal traction as in posterior vitreous detachment (PVD), retinal tear, or retinal detachment.[35,36] Also, patients with migraine (or ocular migraine) might report seeing shimmering arcs of light during the visual aura.[37] Therefore, history of migraine should be ruled out in cases presenting with flashes of light.

Floaters refer to seeing dark spots in the visual field that are caused by vitreous opacities. These opacities could be due to vitreous degeneration with or without PVD, retinal tear, retinal detachment, vitritis as in endophthalmitis, and vitreous hemorrhage as in proliferative diabetic retinopathy.[35,36]

Urgent ophthalmology consultation is mandatory in these cases especially if the flashes and/or floaters are of recent onset and associated with eye pain, eye redness, reduced vision, or visual field deficits.[38]

## Orbital Disorders

### Orbital floor fracture

In these cases, ophthalmology consultation is usually requested after stabilizing the patients and obtaining the standard imaging protocol in trauma patients. Although CT scan is the standard imaging modality for diagnosing orbital floor fracture,[39] it does not replace careful history or a basic eye examination by the admitting provider. History taking should include mode of injury, vision changes, double vision, and eye pain. All parts of the basic eye examination are important in these cases. Special consideration should be given to the globe position, contour, symmetry between both globes, pupil examination, and extraocular movement with special attention to any sign of oculocardiac reflex (bradycardia or hypotension with eye movement).[40]

### Orbital cellulitis

Orbital cellulitis most commonly occurs when bacterial infection spreads from the paranasal sinuses. It is a sight-threatening infection that might be sometimes difficult to differentiate from preseptal cellulitis. The presence of vision changes, proptosis, external ophthalmoplegia, and pupillary abnormalities suggests orbital cellulitis. CT scan of the orbit is important in identifying the extension of the cellulitis and the presence of any abscesses or sinus disease. The most common organisms in orbital cellulitis are usually gram-positive cocci like streptococci.[41] However, in immunocompromised patients as in poorly controlled diabetics with diabetic ketoacidosis, malignancies such as leukemia and lymphoma, mucormycosis might be the causative organism. It is an aggressive opportunistic fungal rhino-orbital infection with poor prognosis and high risk of morbidity and mortality. Symptoms are consistent with eyelid and facial swelling, acute or chronic sinusitis; blood-tinged secretions; headaches; fever; and malaise in an immunocompromised patient. Direct visualization of the palate or nasal mucosa and paranasal sinuses can reveal dark, necrotic tissue and a characteristic black eschar, which results from vascular invasion and tissue infarction.[42]

## Inpatient Screening Eye Examination

Screening examinations constitute a significant number of inpatient ophthalmic consultations.[1–3,43] Screening for papilledema and endogenous endophthalmitis in septicemia or fungemia is a common consultation request for the inpatient ophthalmology service.

### Papilledema

Papilledema is swelling of optic nerve head owing to elevated intracranial pressure.[44] The inpatient team usually requests ophthalmic consultation to either confirm or rule out optic nerve head swelling to assist in the evaluation of cases with suspected intracranial hypertension. The presence of optic nerve head swelling in a patient with headache is highly suggestive of elevated intracranial pressure; however, it is important to highlight that patients may have elevated intracranial pressure without apparent optic nerve head swelling.[45] Therefore, ophthalmology evaluation in these cases should be interpreted within the context of the overall clinical picture of the patient.

### Endogenous endophthalmitis

Endogenous endophthalmitis occurs in less than 0.04% of patients with bacteremia and 0.5% of patients with fungemia.[46] However, it is a common reason for inpatient ophthalmic consultation. Endogenous endophthalmitis can be asymptomatic[47] or present with eye pain, red eye, blurry vision, and floaters.[48] The risk is higher in patients with longer hospital stay, HIV infection, endocarditis, meningitis, lymphoma or leukemia, and abscess of an organ or joint.[46] The most common cause of bacterial endogenous endophthalmitis is gram-positive bacteria, especially methicillin-resistant *Staphylococcus aureus*.[9,46,47] Candida is the most common fungal cause of endogenous endophthalmitis.[46] Current guidelines strongly recommend continuing the current practice of requesting ophthalmic evaluation in all patients with fungemia given the subtle presentation in some cases.[3,49,50]

## CLINICS CARE POINTS

---

- Patients might have intracranial hypertension with no papilledema on fundus examination.
- Ophthalmology consultation is warranted for all inpatients with fungemia even if the patients have no eye symptoms.

---

## SUMMARY

Inpatients might present with a broad spectrum of ocular disorders that have variable levels of acuity. Obtaining a detailed history and performing a basic eye examination by the inpatient provider are a key step in triaging these conditions. In general, ophthalmic consultation should be obtained in all patients presenting with sudden loss or decrease of vision, sudden onset of visual field deficit, flashes/floaters, and severe eye pain especially if associated with vision changes. Advanced in imaging and health care delivery with remote imaging and teleophthalmology may help improve the delivery of ophthalmic care to hospitals without an active inpatient ophthalmology consult service. Clear communication between the inpatient and ophthalmology teams is critical for delivery of optimum eye care to the inpatients presenting with eye complaints.

## CONFLICT OF INTEREST

No conflicting relationship exists for any author.

## REFERENCES

1. Carter K, Miller KM. Ophthalmology inpatient consultation. Ophthalmology 2001; 108(8):1505–11.
2. Grewal DS, Chiang E, Wong E, et al. Adult ophthalmology inpatient consults at a tertiary care teaching hospital. Ophthalmology 2014;121(7):1489–91.e1481.
3. Oh DJ, Kanu LN, Chen JL, et al. Inpatient and emergency room ophthalmology consultations at a tertiary care center. J Ophthalmol 2019;2019:7807391.
4. Kang HK, Luff AJ. Management of retinal detachment: a guide for non-ophthalmologists. BMJ 2008;336(7655):1235–40.
5. Kedar S, Ghate D, Corbett JJ. Visual fields in neuro-ophthalmology. Indian J Ophthalmol 2011;59(2):103–9.
6. Wilhelm H. Disorders of the pupil. Handb Clin Neurol 2011;102:427–66.
7. Enyedi LB, Dev S, Cox TA. A comparison of the Marcus Gunn and alternating light tests for afferent pupillary defects. Ophthalmology 1998;105(5):871–3.
8. Shingleton BJ, O'Donoghue MW. Blurred vision. N Engl J Med 2000;343(8): 556–62.
9. Wu ZH, Chan RP, Luk FO, et al. Review of clinical features, microbiological spectrum, and treatment outcomes of endogenous endophthalmitis over an 8-year period. J Ophthalmol 2012;2012:265078.
10. Chen JJ, Bhatti MT. Papilledema. Int Ophthalmol Clin 2019;59(3):3–22.
11. Pula JH, Kwan K, Yuen CA, et al. Update on the evaluation of transient vision loss. Clin Ophthalmol 2016;10:297–303.
12. Paul NL, Simoni M, Rothwell PM. Transient isolated brainstem symptoms preceding posterior circulation stroke: a population-based study. Lancet Neurol 2013; 12(1):65–71.
13. The International Classification of Headache Disorders: 2nd edition. Cephalalgia 2004;24(Suppl 1):9–160.
14. Spraul CW, Grossniklaus HE. Vitreous hemorrhage. Surv Ophthalmol 1997; 42(1):3–39.
15. Bagheri N, Mehta S. Acute vision loss. Prim Care Clin Office Pract 2015;42(3): 347–61.
16. Rodrigues EB, Penha FM, Melo GB, et al. CHAPTER 15 - Retina and ocular toxicity to ocular application of drugs. In: Nguyen QD, Rodrigues EB, Farah ME, et al, editors. Retinal pharmacotherapy. Edinburgh (Scotland): W.B. Saunders; 2010. p. 96–103.
17. Hsien YM, Mustapha M, Hamzah JC, et al. Why can't I see after my heart is fixed: a case series of ocular complications after cardiac intervention. BMC Ophthalmol 2016;16(1):32.
18. Byrd S, Hussaini AS, Antisdel J. Acute vision loss following endoscopic sinus surgery. Case Rep Otolaryngol 2017;2017:4935123.
19. Leibowitz HM. The red eye. N Engl J Med 2000;343(5):345–51.
20. Dunlop AL, Wells JR. Approach to red eye for primary care practitioners. Prim Care 2015;42(3):267–84.

21. Akpek EK, Uy HS, Christen W, et al. Severity of episcleritis and systemic disease association. Ophthalmology 1999;106(4):729–31.
22. Sainz de la Maza M, Molina N, Gonzalez-Gonzalez LA, et al. Clinical characteristics of a large cohort of patients with scleritis and episcleritis. Ophthalmology 2012;119(1):43–50.
23. Albini TA, Rao NA, Smith RE. The diagnosis and management of anterior scleritis. Int Ophthalmol Clin 2005;45(2):191–204.
24. Bourcier T, Thomas F, Borderie V, et al. Bacterial keratitis: predisposing factors, clinical and microbiological review of 300 cases. Br J Ophthalmol 2003;87(7): 834–8.
25. Rosenbaum JT, Lin P, Asquith M. Does the microbiome cause B27-related acute anterior uveitis? Ocul Immunol Inflamm 2016;24(4):440–4.
26. Connell PP, O'Neill EC, Fabinyi D, et al. Endogenous endophthalmitis: 10-year experience at a tertiary referral centre. Eye (Lond). 2011;25(1):66–72.
27. Chaudhry IA, Shamsi FA, Elzaridi E, et al. Outcome of treated orbital cellulitis in a tertiary eye care center in the Middle East. Ophthalmology 2007;114(2):345–54.
28. Sagiv O, Thakar SD, Kandl TJ, et al. Clinical course of preseptal and orbital cellulitis in 50 immunocompromised patients with cancer. Ophthalmology 2018; 125(2):318–20.
29. Liu Y, Lobo AM, Sobrin L. Endophthalmitis in immunocompromised and diabetic patients. In: Durand M, Miller J, Young L, editors. Endophthalmitis. Springer, Cham. 2016. p. 223–8. https://doi.org/10.1007/978-3-319-29231-1_13.
30. Pflipsen M, Massaquoi M, Wolf S. Evaluation of the painful eye. Am Fam Physician 2016;93(12):991–8.
31. Shields T, Sloane PD. A comparison of eye problems in primary care and ophthalmology practices. Fam Med 1991;23(7):544–6.
32. Nash EA, Margo CE. Patterns of emergency department visits for disorders of the eye and ocular adnexa. Arch Ophthalmol 1998;116(9):1222–6.
33. Halilovic EA, Alimanovic I, Suljic E, et al. Optic neuritis as first clinical manifestations the multiple sclerosis. Mater Sociomed 2014;26(4):246–8.
34. Munir SZ, Aylward J. A review of ocular graft-versus-host disease. Optom Vis Sci 2017;94(5):545–55.
35. Johnson D, Hollands H. Acute-onset floaters and flashes. CMAJ 2012;184(4):431.
36. Sharma P, Sridhar J, Mehta S. Flashes and floaters. Prim Care Clin Office Pract 2015;42(3):425–35.
37. Arunagiri G, Santhi S. Migraine: an ophthalmologist's perspective. Curr Opin Ophthalmol 2003;14(6):344–52.
38. Kahawita S, Simon S, Gilhotra J. Flashes and floaters—a practical approach to assessment and management. Aust Fam Physician 2014;43:201–3.
39. Boyette JR, Pemberton JD, Bonilla-Velez J. Management of orbital fractures: challenges and solutions. Clin Ophthalmol 2015;9:2127–37.
40. Pham CM, Couch SM. Oculocardiac reflex elicited by orbital floor fracture and inferior globe displacement. Am J Ophthalmol Case Rep 2017;6:4–6.
41. Tsirouki T, Dastiridou AI, Ibánez Flores N, et al. Orbital cellulitis. Surv Ophthalmol 2018;63(4):534–53.
42. Roden MM, Zaoutis TE, Buchanan WL, et al. Epidemiology and outcome of zygomycosis: a review of 929 reported cases. Clin Infect Dis 2005;41(5):634–53.
43. Rizzuti AE, Vastardi M, Hajee M, et al. Scope of resident ophthalmology consultation service and patient follow-up rates at a level 1 trauma center in Brooklyn, New York. Clin Ophthalmol 2013;7:643–7.

44. Rigi M, Almarzouqi SJ, Morgan ML, et al. Papilledema: epidemiology, etiology, and clinical management. Eye Brain 2015;7:47–57.
45. Friedman DI, Liu GT, Digre KB. Revised diagnostic criteria for the pseudotumor cerebri syndrome in adults and children. Neurology 2013;81(13):1159–65.
46. Vaziri K, Pershing S, Albini TA, et al. Risk factors predictive of endogenous endophthalmitis among hospitalized patients with hematogenous infections in the United States. Am J Ophthalmol 2015;159(3):498–504.
47. Wang K, Krishnan G, Pershing S. Ophthalmology consultation to detect endogenous endophthalmitis: clinical characteristics in consulted versus diagnosed cases among at-risk inpatients. Ophthalmic Surg Lasers Imaging Retina 2020; 51(3). 159-a153.
48. Jackson TL, Eykyn SJ, Graham EM, et al. Endogenous bacterial endophthalmitis: a 17-year prospective series and review of 267 reported cases. Surv Ophthalmol 2003;48(4):403–23.
49. Adam MK, Vahedi S, Nichols MM, et al. Inpatient ophthalmology consultation for fungemia: prevalence of ocular involvement and necessity of funduscopic screening. Am J Ophthalmol 2015;160(5):1078–83.e1072.
50. Pappas PG, Kauffman CA, Andes DR, et al. Clinical practice guideline for the management of candidiasis: 2016 update by the Infectious Diseases Society of America. Clin Infect Dis 2016;62(4):e1–50.

# Moving?

## Make sure your subscription moves with you!

To notify us of your new address, find your **Clinics Account Number** (located on your mailing label above your name), and contact customer service at:

**Email: journalscustomerservice-usa@elsevier.com**

**800-654-2452** (subscribers in the U.S. & Canada)
**314-447-8871** (subscribers outside of the U.S. & Canada)

**Fax number: 314-447-8029**

**Elsevier Health Sciences Division**
**Subscription Customer Service**
**3251 Riverport Lane**
**Maryland Heights, MO 63043**

*To ensure uninterrupted delivery of your subscription, please notify us at least 4 weeks in advance of move.

# Moving?

## Make sure your subscription moves with you!

To notify us of your new address, find your Clinics Account Number (located on your mailing label above your name), and contact customer service at:

Email: journalscustomerservice-usa@elsevier.com

800-654-2452 (subscribers in the U.S. & Canada)
314-447-8871 (subscribers outside of the U.S. & Canada)

Fax number: 314-447-8029

Elsevier Health Sciences Division
Subscription Customer Service
3251 Riverport Lane
Maryland Heights, MO 63043